Managing Stress in the Christian Family

Jere L. Phillips, PhD

Foreword by James Klemis, MD, FACC, FSCAI

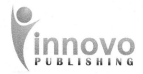

Published by
Innovo Publishing, LLC
www.innovopublishing.com
1-888-546-2111

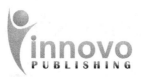

Providing Full-Service Publishing Services for
Christian Authors, Artists & Organizations: Hardbacks, Paperbacks,
eBooks, Audiobooks, Music & Film

MANAGING STRESS IN THE CHRISTIAN FAMILY
Copyright © 2016 Jere L. Phillips, PhD
All rights reserved.

Unless otherwise indicated, Scripture is taken from the Holy Bible King James Version. Note: Author has changed some wording, such as "thee" and "ye" to "you," for ease of reading.

Library of Congress Control Number: 2016938111
ISBN: 978-1-61314-280-6

Cover Design & Interior Layout: Innovo Publishing, LLC

Printed in the United States of America
U.S. Printing History
First Edition: May 2016

ABOUT THE AUTHOR

Dr. Jere Phillips has been helping people for over forty years. In personal counseling, teaching, and writing, he has shared biblical truths that people of all ages can implement effectively. His study of stress began with a life-threatening, stress-related illness. He soon was asked by families in his church to share what he had learned. These principles have been taught in colleges and churches. Groups have included health-care professionals, pastors, and Christian families. He has published in a wide variety of subjects and venues, including an article on managing stress in *Departure* magazine—a journal for professional travelers.

His first book, *The Missionary Family: Managing Stress Effectively*, provided some of the foundational ideas for this current work. His second book is *Pastoral Ministry for the Next Generation*. Phillips holds a PhD degree from New Orleans Baptist Theological Seminary with a major in preaching and a minor in psychology and counseling. Currently he is Professor of Practical Theology at Mid-America Baptist Theological Seminary. He and his wife, Glenda, have two married children and seven grandchildren.

WHAT OTHERS SAY ABOUT THIS BOOK:

"Through an examination of Scripture enhanced by a scientific understanding of God's design in people, Jere Phillips' *Managing Stress in the Christian Family* provides a comprehensive and practical guide to understanding and biblically dealing with stress across every phase of life."
—Joshua A. Creason, PhD

"Jere Phillips writes from both educational and experiential background in his book, *Managing Stress in the Christian Family*. Stress is a sometimes visitor to every family on earth regardless of whether the family is Christian. However, as is sometimes the case, some Christian families feel being Christian protects them from stress. On the contrary, as Dr. Phillips points out, Christian families have the extra burden of modeling managing stress. Not simply a tool, the book is a nuts and bolts example of structuring life under the safe keeping of God's grace so that the Holy Spirit offers solutions and not simply descriptions of problems. Every caregiver who works with families will need a copy."
—Dr. Brooks Faulkner, Lifeway Christian Resources, retired

"Taking care of our bodies physically, emotionally, and spiritually can allow us to have the peace in our lives that Jesus promised. We will not experience the absence of stress, but we can learn how to deal with the inevitable stressors of life in a way that we aren't consumed by them. These concepts are something we can learn from this book as we look toward the counsel of the Great Physician Himself."
—James Klemis, MD FACC FSCAI

"I see the effects of stress in my medical practice on an almost daily basis. While there is no simple 'recipe' that solves all such problems, it seems to me that a balanced approach is what is missing the most. The medical profession (and psychiatrists) tend to think of stress as a serotonin-mediated problem that can be reduced to, and altered by, chemical intervention. I believe there is value in that approach but not exclusively. I find chapter 5—dealing with methods for stress management—particularly beneficial, especially in a world that is looking for 'relief in a bottle.'"
—David Ball, MD

CONTENTS

Foreword by James Klemis, MD, FACC, FSCAI

Preface: I Nearly Died—Twice!

1. All God's Families Have Problems 17
    Challenges in the Christian Family

2. So, What Is Stress Anyway? 31
    Understanding the Nature of Stress

3. Where Does Stress Come From?..47
    Sources of Stress

4. How Can Stress Affect My Life?...63
    Evidence of Unmanaged Stress

5. So What Do I Do About It?...75
    Methods for Managing Stress

6. What Else Can I Do to Help My Marriage and Family?....................107
    Marriage and Family Issues

7. Who Will Take Care of Me? 121
    Help for Caregivers

8. What's the Problem? 133
    Reducing Stress through Conflict Resolution

9. What about the Giants in My Life? 153
    Handling Bullies

10. What about Special Cases? 165
    Extreme Stress: Burnout and PTSD

Conclusion: HOPE!...173

Endnotes 175

Bibliography..179

FOREWORD

By James Klemis, MD, FACC, FSCAI
Interventional Cardiology
Stern Cardiovascular Foundation
Memphis, TN

I came to know the author of this book during a stressful period in his life—I was his doctor when he presented with a massive heart attack. Thankfully we were able to open the blocked artery and he survived the event. He has recovered and led a fairly active life since. We see each other in the office for routine checkups, and I was asked to write the foreword to this book during a recent visit.

As a physician and interventional cardiologist, I have studied the physiological effects of stress on the human body and mind. I have been with patients and families during extremely stressful periods in their lives. I experience stress to a degree when I am in the middle of a complex procedure and have the responsibility of caring for patients. There are positive and negative aspects of stress. Our body's "fight or flight" response can use stress to sharpen our senses and help us to react in a way that can get us out of harm.

In some conditions, extremely stressful situations can be harmful. In many medical conditions, the body can be overwhelmed by stress, causing real emotional or physical issues. Takotsubo cardiomyopathy is one condition that comes to mind. Usually seen among female patients who have a sudden severe stressful issue, it can mimic a heart attack exactly, shows the same changes on an EKG, and causes the same damage to the heart muscle that we see from a blocked artery (although during the coronary angiogram we see normal blood flow in the arteries). Thankfully, these patients tend to recover by placing them on a medication called a beta blocker, which blocks the harmful effects of the body's stress chemicals on the heart.

All of us will experience stress during our lives, not only in the medical/physical realm, but in the day-to-day issues we face at work, in our family relationships, and in our social lives. Often the stress is due to situations beyond our control and can lead to hopelessness and despair. In John 16:33, Jesus said, "These things I have spoken unto you, that in me ye might have peace. In the world ye shall have tribulation: but be of good cheer; I have overcome the world." He didn't promise a stress-free life but did promise He would give us His peace, even in stressful situations.

The Caduceus is the symbol for medicine. It shows a snake wrapped around a staff. The symbolism reflects a famous passage in the book of Numbers in which the Israelites were in the desert being attacked by snakes. God told Moses to lift up his staff with the bronze serpent and whoever looked at it would be healed. Jesus referenced this same passage when He said, "And as Moses lifted up the serpent in the wilderness, even so must the Son of man be lifted up, that whosoever believeth in him should not perish, but have eternal life" (John 3:14–15). The significance to me is that God doesn't always remove us from stressful situations or environments (the Israelites had actually prayed for God to remove the snakes) but may use them to cause us to turn to Him in faith.

Managing stress is an important part of our physical, emotional, and spiritual health. As a physician, part of my job is to make an appropriate diagnosis of my patient's condition and then prescribe a treatment plan to manage the condition and allow the patient to get well. Either wrong diagnoses or wrong treatments can be harmful. In the same way, we need guidelines in our lives to help us deal with stress.

The apostle Paul had a time in his life when he was dealing with incredible difficulty and said, "For this thing I besought the Lord three times, that it might depart from me, And he said unto me, My grace is sufficient for thee: for my strength is made perfect in weakness. Most gladly therefore will I rather glory in my infirmities, that the power of Christ may rest upon me" (2 Corinthians 12:8–9). Once again, we see that Paul prayed for God to remove the stress, but instead God had a different plan that was better. Paul had a correct diagnosis, but God had a better treatment plan.

Taking care of our bodies physically, emotionally, and spiritually can allow us to have the peace in our lives that Jesus promised. We will not experience the absence of stress, but we can learn how to deal with the inevitable stressors of life in a way that we aren't consumed by them. Too, we can learn to have peace in our lives even in the midst of stress. These concepts are something I think we can learn from this book as we look toward the counsel of the "Great Physician" Himself.

Preface

I NEARLY DIED—TWICE!

I nearly died in 1979 from a rare combination of several stress-related diseases. Surviving by the grace of God, I began studying the nature of stress, its causes, effects, and treatments. Most of the material dealt with the medical and psychological aspects, but none mentioned the spiritual nature of stress management, nor did any of the works address the cross-linking of various causes, effects, and treatments.

As a result of my work, and at the request of church members who heard about my experience and studies, I developed a Christian Stress Management workshop that included many of the principles found in these pages. This workshop was presented in churches, a local college, and even at an association of medical workers. I published an article in *Departure* (a magazine for professional travelers) under the title "Overcoming the Traveler's #1 Enemy: Stress."

After a few years, however, I shelved the material and did not think about it for many years, until I nearly died again thirty years later in 2009, this time of a massive heart attack. God used a godly cardiologist to save my life. I remain ever grateful to the Lord and to that physician, Dr. James Klemis, who wrote the foreword to this book.

During the intervening years, I was blessed to serve as a pastor and church staff member, a missions administrator in two state conventions (Director of the Missions Department for the Tennessee Baptist Convention and Executive Director for the West Virginia Convention of Southern Baptists), and as interim pastor in over fifteen churches. God also has allowed me to travel to countries on six continents on nearly thirty short-term mission trips.

Over those years, I counseled with countless individuals, married couples, and families. They have had problems that filled the widest range of issues you might imagine. Usually, their difficulties included at least two primary issues: sin and stress. In the first case, the issue is basic: confess and repent of the sin and seek God's forgiveness and restoration. However, stress was not always so easily identifiable since it masqueraded as so many symptoms—conflict in marriages, struggles at work, rebellion among teenagers, substance abuse, anxiety, fear, and much more.

I did not revisit my previous work in stress management until a regional conference of the Evangelical Missiological Society issued a call for papers regarding missionary families and their well-being. I found it necessary to restudy much of my previous work with investigation into more recent works and a much deeper study of God's Word than before.

After presenting a small paper on this subject at the conference, several people encouraged me to develop it into a book, which was published in 2013—*The Missionary Family: Managing Stress Effectively*. It was well received, but it led to the question: What about the average Christian family? Can we offer solid biblical and practical help for them?

This book was not written from a desire to be published; I have already published two major books (*The Missionary Family: Managing Stress Effectively* and *Pastoral Ministry for the Next Generation*) and five smaller ones, along with over two hundred articles and lessons whose total circulation exceeded 20 million. Rather, this work has the specific prayer that it will help your family (and mine!) overcome the daily pressures that diminish your effectiveness in the home, at work and school, and among your neighbors in the community at large.

A shortcut through these pages would simply bring you to Jesus, for He alone gives peace: "Peace I leave with you, my peace I give unto you: not as the world gives, give I unto you. Let not your heart be troubled, neither let it be afraid" (John 14:27). Any lasting solution for life and work must be found in Christ. These few pages have one goal—to point readers to the One Who can strengthen them and enable them to overcome the stressors they encounter.

This book features three distinctive approaches:

1. **It addresses the entire family.** Each member of the family has special needs and encounters unique stressors. Prayerfully they all will find help in this volume. **Notice to single adults**: Families come in all shapes and sizes. A family of one, the single adult, can find help in this volume. Every person can discover principles that touch real life.

2. **It builds on the Word of God.** This book finds its basis of truth (its epistemology) in Scripture alone. Throughout the work, you will see biblical references. These notations are not merely offered as proof-texts, but are provided with the hope you will open the Bible and read along. Only God's Spirit through God's Word can bring you to God's Son. He is the answer for all our needs, including handling the stressors of life.

3. **It integrates causes, effects, and management methods with the five parts of human nature**—the spirit, the body, and the soul (the soul includes our mind, will, emotions). One cannot separate the various elements of the human composition, for we are integrated, whole persons. Each area of the human being corresponds to various causes, effects, and management methods, which relate specifically to that area. At the same time, each part of a person affects each other part. Thus, a spiritual cause may have a physical effect. An emotional effect may have a management method related to the mind. So, this work attempts to integrate each of these areas as much as possible within our limitations.

Special Note: The examples found in this work represent composites of situations people experience. Names, locations, and other details have been changed so no individual might be identified with any portrayal. In addition, the writer does not claim to offer psychological counsel or medical advice. This book involves spiritual and practical observations based on Scripture, research, and experience. People suffering from severe stress should consult appropriate medical professionals.

Chapter One

ALL GOD'S FAMILIES HAVE PROBLEMS

Challenges in the Christian Family

When the phone rings at three in the morning, it is never good news. Pastor Jim[1] shook himself awake and answered, readying himself for whatever crisis had jarred him from sleep. The shaking voice said, "Fred killed himself." Pastor Jim was stunned. Fred had been a strong member of his church—a seemingly successful businessman, faithful husband, and good father. While Jim quickly dressed to go and help this grief-stricken family, he wondered, "What could have driven Fred to take his own life?"

As Fred's story unfolded over the next two days, Pastor Jim learned that Fred had been experiencing a perfect storm of several serious problems. Seeking help would have required admission of the problem and facing his friends and family with what he viewed as unacceptable failure. Instead, he fled in the most extreme way possible. The stress of his situation had produced so much emotional pain that he believed he had only one option for escape.

Lest a reader jump to the conclusion that you know who this is, you don't. I know of over half a dozen situations in which this scenario played out with problems ranging from finances to long-term physical illnesses to depression. Each one left a grieving family broken over an act of desperation.

Every day, usually in less dramatic circumstances, families suffer from the pressures of life. Most people cope with various levels of success, usually managing to work past the immediate stress and experiencing some degree of normality. Yet, every person, even Christians, have burdens to bear and problems to solve.

No One Is Exempt from Stress

Some people think being a Christian means not having problems or stress. They believe that when you are saved God wipes out every worry and calms every fear. Certainly God can do that, but the Bible also addresses many situations in which Christians suffer, engage in conflict, are persecuted, or experience personal difficulties.

Christians are not immune to the stressors of life. In the workplace, they have deadlines to meet, bills to pay, and children to raise. Teenagers wrestle with the usual conflicting dynamics of changing hormones, peer pressure, and developmental crises. Children go through the stress of starting and staying in school, learning to handle group interactions, and coping with family issues. All of us have problems and each one involves some level of stress.

Stress is not uniquely exclusive to conflict or pressures. Every change in life involves some degree of stress. We'll talk more about the nature of stress in the next chapter. At this point, we need to realize stress is a normal part of life, even in the Christian family. The focus of this book is not how to eliminate stress from your life. That's impossible! We cannot totally escape stress, but we can learn to manage our reaction to it. Through Christ, we can overcome the debilitating effects of stress and live victorious lives.

Consider How Stress Can Affect Family Members at All Stages of Life

1. **Following Paul's footsteps—the problems and possibilities of singleness**

The first unit of the family is the individual. Some individuals marry other individuals. Most individuals who marry have children, who are also individuals. My redundant point is that our concept of the family begins with each person, including those people who remain single—whether for a period of time or for a lifetime. Once individuals marry, they are no longer simply individuals; the two have become one flesh (Genesis 2:23; Matthew 19:6). Still, we need to recognize that principles relating to managing stress in the Christian family apply to unmarried adults as well as to people who are married.

Other than Jesus, the most famous single adult in Scripture was the apostle Paul. Some commentators think Paul may have been a widower, but nothing in the Bible suggests he was ever married. In fact, Paul thought believers would be better off if they remained unmarried so they could give total attention to their service to Christ (1 Corinthians 7:6–9, 32–34). Singleness can offer wonderful possibilities for serving the Lord without the distraction of other concerns. Yet, it comes with additional complications.

Single people experience many of the same stressors that married families have, but they also deal with problems unique to being single. Paul recognized that not every person was called to a life of single celibacy and encouraged people to marry if they could not handle the stress of life without sexual intimacy (1 Corinthians 7:9). **Managing sexual urges** is one of the most difficult sources of stress in the single person's life. The Holy Spirit can empower Christian singles to resist temptation and happily live chaste lives of holiness.

Additional areas of stress for the single adult include the following:

The need for companionship. Certainly, singles can find a level of companionship at church, in the workplace, at social events, and in normal friendships. However, none of these options substitute for the desire for more intimate, permanent companionship with someone who is present in one's life day after day. While the church is not a matchmaker venue, it should be intentional in providing genuine *koinonia* (godly fellowship) for all members, including single adults.

Financial challenges create another area of stress. Married couples often have supplemental income when both spouses work. Having dual incomes provides additional resources for the family as well as some level of security in case one or the other loses a job. Single adults lack this advantage. While their expenses are usually less than that of a married family with children, their financial needs can exert significant stress.

The desire for children. Most people, females perhaps more so than males, have an inner need to procreate, to have a child to nourish and love. Single adults find the frustration of this need stressful. Many states now allow single adults to adopt children, which is one solution. However, the longing of a woman to bear a child of her own cannot be underestimated.

2. Marriage is messy and marvelous

Scripture places a high value on marriage. The first wedding occurred in the Garden of Eden when God created the woman from the side of the man and brought them together as husband and wife (Genesis 2:24–25). Although He remained a single adult, Jesus blessed marriage by being present at a wedding in Cana of Galilee (John 2:1–2). As we have mentioned, Paul recognized the value of remaining single, but at the same time he wrote, ". . . let every man have his own wife and let every woman have her own husband" (1 Corinthians 7:2).

Having been married for forty-four years at the time of this writing, let me testify that marriage is a wonderful blessing from God. No other relationship in life is like that created when a man and woman fully give themselves to the Lord, Who gives them to one another in marriage. Yet each aspect of blessing has challenges that can involve stress if both parties do not live out biblical principles related to their relationship. Consider a few of these issues:

A lifelong commitment. The basic building block of the Christian family is a man and woman committed to each other until death alone parts them. Modern ideas of serial monogamy, open marriage, and trial marriages are foreign to God's Word and destructive to the family. Jesus reminded His disciples that divorce was not part of God's plan, but from the beginning the Lord intended the marriage relationship to last for a lifetime (Matthew 19:4–6).

At the same time, a lifetime together can produce its own stressful situation unless the man and woman follow the biblical model for a godly marriage. As they grow older, many of the factors that drew them to one another change. They may not look as attractive as during their courtship. Their communication might wear thin. Habits that were overlooked become more irritating as time goes by. None of these and other issues should offer the slightest basis for ending the relationship.

Rather, every problem provides an opportunity for the couple to explore their marriage and find ways to strengthen and deepen their relationship.

Sexual intimacy. Scripture has much to say about human sexuality. However, many couples have not been properly instructed as to what the Bible has to say about a healthy sexual relationship. Consequently, they may struggle in this important area of life. Instead of being satisfying and deepening their union, immature sexuality can become a major source of stress in the marriage.

Worldly approaches to sexuality add to the harmful ways many husbands and wives respond to sexual stress. Men may begin viewing pornography. Increasingly, women are also drawn to illicit online voyeurism. Couples who take each other for granted, both sexually and in other ways, may become tempted to gratify themselves with relationships outside of their marriage. Problems can also develop if either party sees sex as a way simply to meet their own needs rather than giving pleasure to the spouse.

While we will address some of these issues in a later chapter, consider a few biblical principles that help solve some of the sexual difficulties couples encounter. Scripture encourages married couples to maintain consistent sexual intimacy to avoid the temptations of the devil (1 Corinthians 7:5). The husband and wife are reminded that in marriage their bodies are given to each other willingly and joyfully (1 Corinthians 7:4). The Bible reminds us that "the marriage bed" should be "kept undefiled." Therefore the husband and wife must maintain their exclusive commitment to one another and reject "immoral people" who would tempt them to betray their spouses (Hebrews 13:4).

Decision making. Who gets to decide both small and great matters in the home? One of the prime factors in most divorces relates to the struggle for control in the marriage. Even Christian families often misunderstand what it means for the husband to be the head of the household. Many people emphasize the commandment for wives to submit themselves to their husbands, but most misunderstand the full context of Paul's admonition.

The primary passage relating to decision making is Ephesians 5:21–25. Notice that before telling the wives to submit to their husbands, Paul encouraged everyone to submit to one another in the fear of God (verse 21).

When believing spouses have the servant spirit that Christ exemplified, they will set aside personal needs to minister to one another (see John 13:12–17).

Notice, too, the wives are to submit to their "own husbands"—a clear instruction to be faithful to their husbands. This submission is to be "as unto the Lord," meaning the way in which they relate to their husbands is as if they were serving Christ. Similarly, the husband should love his wife sacrificially, as Christ lovingly gave Himself for us (Ephesians 5:25).

When husbands and wives have this kind of servant attitude toward one another the tug of war over decisions ends. Each person works to find the solution that honors the Lord and benefits one another.

3. Parenting isn't for sissies.

Being a parent is one of the most blessed facets of life and, at the same time, produces some of the most stressful aspects of family life. Children are a blessing from God (Psalm 127:3–5), but raising children requires strength that comes from God alone. Each life brought into the world comes from Him and should be cherished as a gift from God. Still, bearing and raising children involve stresses that change with every phase of development.

As Hannah with Samuel and Mary with Jesus, parents begin well by dedicating each child to the Lord (1 Samuel 1:19–28; Luke 2:22–24). By His grace and with His aid, parents can overcome all challenges and rejoice to see His hand in their children's lives.

Bearing Children. Becoming a parent is full of happiness and anticipation, but it also creates numerous sources of stress. The physical changes in a woman's body can be both joyous (knowing she bears another life within her) and stressful. Weight gain, the need for maternity clothes, painful ankles, and many other issues produce daily stress. Effects of hormonal change can throw both the woman and her husband into a roller coaster of emotions. Couples need to get good information about what to expect and how to respond to each phase of pregnancy.

Some pregnancies end in miscarriage. Numerous causes may result in the placenta separating from the womb, or the child dying before birth, or some other problem that ends the pregnancy. The mother and father grieve at the loss of a baby they never got to know. In some cases, the woman may become unable to bear children, adding to the extreme stress of the tragedy. Relatives, friends, and church associates can offer comfort and support, but no one should underestimate the emotional toll on the parents.

Adoption. Some couples are not able to conceive children of their own. Hannah, who eventually became the mother of the prophet Samuel, was unable to have children for many years. She pleaded with the Lord for a child (1 Samuel 1:27). The frustration of wanting children but being unable to have them can be heartbreakingly stressful. One couple tried numerous doctors, paid for countless procedures, and endured failure after failure. Denial is one of the normal stages of grief, and they refused to consider adoption for many years, thinking that to do so would be a lack of faith that God would hear their prayers. Finally, they received peace from the Lord that they could indeed have a child, but He would provide one through adoption. Once they completed the process, they praised God for His goodness and embraced their adopted child wholeheartedly.

Adoption is a blessing to the parents and the children. Adopted children should never feel less loved because they grew up in adoptive homes. Moses was adopted (Exodus 2:5–10), as was Esther (Esther 2:7). The Bible uses the picture of adoption to describe believers' relationship with our heavenly Father Who adopts us through the redemption made possible by Christ (Romans 8:14–17).

A family adopts a child to offer hope and happiness as well as a home. Our youngest daughter already had three biological children when she and her husband adopted a special needs child from China. During a trip while in college, she discovered the dire situation many babies, especially female infants, faced. Years later, she and her husband sacrificed in many ways to bring one of those babies into our family. This child receives as much love and acceptance as any of the other children and remains a joy to us all.

Still, adoption has its challenges. Financially, the adoptive family discovers the process is expensive and requires extensive time and effort. Many families have to travel overseas to find an adoptable child, adding to the strain of the procedure. Emotionally, the child might resist bonding at first. Some adoptive families experience the pain of being rejected by the child they love. Other siblings may struggle with integrating another person into their family. Physically, the adopted child could have medical needs. While families are willing to pay the price to bring these special children into their homes, they need to understand the stress involved and learn how to manage those issues.

Dealing with discipline. No parent enjoys having to discipline a child or teenager. The very act follows a break in trust between parent and child as the child goes against the parent's instruction. Only an ungodly and unloving parent refuses to correct children. Although he was a priest of God, Eli failed to discipline his children and their rebellious wickedness cost them their lives under the judgment of God (1 Samuel 3–4). On the other hand, Proverbs reminds us that a loving parent corrects a child, just as a loving God disciplines us (Proverbs 3:12).

Not only is the act of discipline stressful for parents and children but the manner of correction can also be a source of stress between parents who have different ideas about how to address misbehavior. The father may tend to use corporal punishment, as indicated in Proverbs 19:18: "Chasten thy son while there is hope, and let not thy soul spare for his crying," or Proverbs 29:15: "The rod and reproof give wisdom: but a child left to himself brings his mother to shame." The mother may prefer to focus on discipline through training, as taught in Proverbs 22:6: "Train up a child in the way he should go: and when he is old, he will not depart from it."

Children could avoid discipline by obeying their parents because doing so pleases the Lord. At the same time, Scripture reminds fathers not to "provoke your children to anger, lest they be discouraged" (Colossians 3:20–21).

Favorites. Families invite tension into the home if either parent shows favoritism toward one child versus another. Scripture narrates numerous accounts of the disastrous effects of showing more favor toward one child. Consider the cases of Esau and Jacob (Genesis 25:28), or Jacob and Joseph (Genesis 33:2, 37:3). Feelings of rejection and bitterness can poison any home when children perceive they are not as loved as much as a brother or sister.

Sickness. All children get sick. Some face life-threatening illness or injury. Like Jairus and his daughter (Mark 5:23), parents cannot watch their children suffer without feeling worry and stress. Have you not sat up late at night watching over children aching with fever, bathing their foreheads, and making sure they get medicine? When a parent is stressed over a child's health, nearly everything else becomes secondary. A couple may experience a strain in their relationship as each frets over their child's well-being.

Providing. Putting food on the table and a roof over the family is a normal parental responsibility. Paul reminded Timothy that if anyone did not provide for his own household, he is worse than an unbeliever (1 Timothy 5:8). Stress associated with work can wear on fathers and mothers. When the security of a job is threatened, stress levels rise, along with tempers. Parents can end up acting out their frustrations and fears with harsh words toward one another or their children.

Worry. Most parents worry about their children, even when they grow up and have children of their own. Even Jesus' mother, Mary, was worried when she and Joseph could not find the twelve-year-old (Luke 2:48).

We worry about our children's health, their choices, their friends, their schoolwork, their choice of careers and mates, their mistakes, and their heartaches. Christian parents can reduce their stressful responses by remembering that their children also have a heavenly Father Who cares for them.

My wife and I were in West Virginia some years ago for a major job interview. On the night before the meeting, we called to check on our oldest daughter who was traveling home from college. She told us of an auto accident she had on the interstate. With fear and shock, we first determined she was uninjured, and then told her what to do about the damaged car. As we wept over how close she came to being severely hurt, my first reaction was to turn down the job that would take us so far from her. Then God reminded us that had we been in the car with her, we could not have prevented that accident. We had to trust our daughters into His care. We prayed and gave our girls again to the Lord. With that, we could rest. And so can you!

4. The sweet and sour of childhood

Most people think of childhood as a time of sweetness and innocence. Say the word *children* and images of carefree kids playing and laughing come to mind. That's how childhood ought to be and, thankfully, that's how it is for most children. However, many children grow up in poverty, wondering when, or if, they will get their next meal. Thousands live on the streets with homeless parents or, in some cases, as runaways. Other children live in dysfunctional homes in which one or both parents create such a chaotic, and sometimes dangerous, environment that the child lives in constant fear. Still other children have to take on the role of adult prematurely when being raised by single parents whose work, or personal lives, keeps them away from home, leaving the children to care for themselves or for one another. For such children, stress is a constant companion.

Even in what we might consider to be normal homes, children experience a variety of stressors. Natural developmental issues can put pressure on the children. **Learning to walk and talk** is difficult. Parents may think they are frustrated by not being able to communicate to a preverbal child. Imagine the confusion and exasperation very young children experience by not understanding the world around them, much less being unable to express themselves except by crying.

Another developmental stressor involves **separation anxiety**, especially when the mother tries to leave the child at bedtime or with a baby sitter for the first time. If parents have not worked through this problem, it can become extremely stressful for children when they begin school. Other areas of childhood stress can include **potty training, socialization with other children, normal sibling rivalry, school-related issues,** and **discipline.**

Everyone needs to feel loved, to feel safe, and to understand who they are. Children tend to find their **affirmation, security**, and **identity** wrapped up in their parents. Proverbs 17:6 emphasizes the importance of fathers to children, but the same is true for the mothers. If parents do not understand this need and fail to offer support, the children may feel rejected, fearful, and confused.

5. Teenage trauma and drama

Stress at school is only one aspect of teenage pressures. Certainly, dealing with homework, tests, expectations, socialization, drugs, alcohol, sex, and a plethora of other problems ought to be enough to stress anyone. Some teens perceive minor problems as being much bigger than they are, creating drama whether there is any real trauma or not.

We really need an entire book to consider all the issues teens experience. At this point, be aware of these few examples. They may give us a glimpse into the stressors that teenagers endure.

Physical and emotional changes. Puberty affects the entire person. Physically, hormones involve changes in sexual organs, growth of hair, depth of voice in males, and other issues. Emotionally, male and female teens experience a range of feelings they may be too immature to understand, much less control. Each change produces its own set of stressors.

Social adjustments. Peers become increasingly important to teenagers. They tend to find acceptance and identity from friends, whether at school or church. As teens grow older, school friends have a powerful influence, for good or bad. If students have difficulty fitting in to an appropriate social group, they will seek acceptance from peers who have a negative impact. Parents should not underestimate the power of social stress in their teens' lives. Stronger youths are better capable of withstanding wounding words and personal attacks. Young people who have a more passive personality or who have not had significant nurturing at home will find greater pressure to become like others in their social group.

Identity and independence. A prime source of stress for teenagers is the struggle for individual identity and independence, while at the same time desiring acceptance by social groups that demand conformity. Teens want to discover who they are. Up to this point, they really did not think about personal identity. They were happy to be part of a family. Now they want to establish individuality unique to themselves.

Dating and sexuality. Today's culture puts pressure on young people to become sexually aware and expressive at an increasingly earlier age. Younger teens are not equipped mentally, physically, or emotionally to cope with some of the social expectations produced by media, music, and other powerful forces of a corrupt culture. Wanting to be liked by the opposite sex, teens can feel forced into associations that tempt them to compromise religious teachings and family values. Forming dating relationships and breaking up are cycles that occur many times in teens' development. Each change exerts stress that can be painful.

6. Stress and the senior adult

Once Christians reach their more mature years, most anticipate an easing of life's stress. Images of retirement include days filled with hobbies, travel, or other enjoyable activities followed by relaxing evenings with one's spouse. However, senior years have their unique set of stressors. Here are just a few:

Challenges to values and culture. During their most productive years, adults dominate their culture. They have some level of control over the types of values allowed into their families. The cultural milieu has, to some degree, been fashioned by their generation. As time passes and they grow older, younger generations emerge that refashion culture that is uncomfortable for seniors. Values may conflict in such a way that seniors feel threatened.

One example can be seen in musical worship at church. Every generation loves to sing the style of music they learned as youths. Senior adults can become very uncomfortable when confronted with worship services filled with unfamiliar music accompanied by instruments and rhythms foreign to their own younger days. They may feel they are no longer valued, or that their preferred worship styles are not respected. If the younger generations who often drive the changes in worship do not understand this dynamic and offer some consideration to seniors' desires, the congregation can experience open strife.

Medical issues. As people age, they experience more health-related problems. You can recognize this stage in life when your table discussion eventually gravitates to a comparison of what medication each person is taking. Medical matters are no laughing matter for seniors. They are frustrated that they cannot do everything they once did. Activities become more limited. Doctors' visits become increasingly common.

Fear of infirmity quietly bears upon the minds of people who once assumed they would always enjoy good health. Many seniors experience anxiety over the costs and availability of insurance and quality medical care. Treatments for medical problems can cause tremendous stress.

Financial challenges. Retirement or disability produces financial stress for everyone as advancing age approaches. Many people arrive at the end of their careers without sufficient savings or pensions to supplement governmental safety nets like Social Security. If senior adults do not have a debt-free home, or incur significant health-related costs, they can find themselves living in substandard housing or having to choose between medicine and food. They abandon their idyllic dream of being able to use the freedom of retirement to travel or pursue other activities. Instead, many seniors find themselves searching for jobs, often at the cost of self-respect as well-educated and experienced people end up accepting minimum-wage positions.

Loss of independence. If physical difficulties leave senior adults without the ability to care for themselves, family members may be forced to impose restrictions for the good of their parents. One of the most traumatic experiences is not being able to drive a vehicle. Being dependent on others for transportation reduces a senior to revisiting their childhood when they were unable to determine where and when they could go somewhere.

If families are unable to provide for seniors' physical needs, they may have to make the very difficult decision to place their loved one in a nursing home or assisted care facility. Perhaps one of the most difficult parts of being in the physical care of strangers is the loss of personal dignity, especially if the patient needs care with bowel or bladder problems. The stress is significant, not only for the seniors affected by this condition but for family members who feel they have no other options to care for their aging parents.

Loss of spouse and friends. Death is inevitable for all of us unless Christ returns during our lifetimes. For the believer, far more stressful than one's own death is the loss of one's spouse. I've witnessed many cases in which the death of a husband or wife is followed closely by the death of the spouse, especially in the cases of persons who have been married four or five decades. Suddenly, half of the person is missing.

One friend whose wife died expressed it as not only "the absence of a presence, but the presence of an absence." Since marriage results in two becoming one, death results in the one becoming something less. A huge part of one's life is gone, leaving the survivor wrestling with creating a new kind of life alone. Family members cannot really appreciate the depth of loneliness the death of a spouse creates.

Seniors also begin seeing more and more friends die. Many older adults regularly check the obituary listings in the newspaper to see if anyone they know has died. Since their friends also are in advanced years, such sad discoveries are not unusual, leaving the survivor wondering "Who is next?" Too, the senior adult's social circle is limited at best. When the few remaining long-time friends begin passing on, the loneliness and isolation adds to their load of stress.

So What Do We Do about All This Stress?

This chapter has not been designed to provide all the answers, although hopefully you gained a few insights along the way. Instead, I have tried to outline a number of the kinds of stress that Christian families experience. Only by acknowledging the problem will we begin to seek causes and solutions. Prayerfully, you will begin discovering more specific help in the following chapters. At each step, stop and ask the Holy Spirit to lead you into insight regarding the biblical and practical truths that will help you and your family.

Chapter Two
SO, WHAT IS STRESS ANYWAY?

Understanding the Nature of Stress

Many individuals manage stressors well. Others suffer harmful effects of prolonged, unmanaged stress. Stress rarely reaches the level of threatening one's life, although prolonged unmanaged stress can be a significant contributor to heart disease and stroke. Average people simply allow unmanaged stress to rob them of joy and contentment, raise their blood pressure, goad them into conflicts, and generally make life miserable.

Hans Selye, pioneer in stress management, described stress as the body's reaction to change. Since human beings prefer homeostasis (the status quo), any disruption to the routine produces stress. General Adaptation Syndrome is the term Selye used to describe the body's reaction to change. His theory argues the more life changes one experiences in a short time, the more stress one undergoes.[1]

Psychologists Thomas Holmes and Richard Rahe developed a life-change measurement that assigned incremental points to life changes.[2] However, change alone cannot be a definitive measure of stress. People react differently to various kinds of change. What might be a devastating tragedy to one person might be a welcomed relief to another. For example, Holmes and Rahe place death of a spouse at the top of their stress chart. However, I believe that such loss cannot account in every case for the level of stress assigned to this event. If the deceased were greatly loved and died suddenly or violently, survivors likely would respond with intense grief and experience tremendous stress. On the other hand, if death comes to an older person who had struggled at length with a painful terminal illness, family and friends might feel a sense of relief, knowing their loved one no longer suffers. In the next chapter, we will discuss many of the variables related to individual responses to different stressors.

Stress is not something that happens to people, but involves our reactions to life situations, personal beliefs and attitudes, and relationship issues. People experience stress as a reaction to changing external circumstances, inner conflict, interpersonal relationships, sin, or other influences. Some changes are under our control. We choose to engage in certain behavior that produces various pressures. Other stressors are thrust upon us. Some stress is physiological in nature; at other times, it results from emotional trauma or spiritual failures.

Because human beings are like snowflakes (no two are completely alike), each individual responds differently to diverse stressors. When confronted with various challenges, some people experience varying levels of stress, while others transform the situations into inner motivation for higher achievement.

To grasp concepts regarding stress, we must first apprehend **the nature of the human being.** Too often, counselors treat stressed persons primarily in terms of physical or emotional responses. Psychoanalysts may spend years with a client investigating childhood experiences, dreams, or responses to emotional trauma without approaching the real problems from a biblical position. Physicians often treat sufferers with various medications, attempting to elevate the mood, heal an ulcer, or moderate the blood pressure. Doctors rarely have the luxury of enough time to engage their patients in lengthy discussions about their life circumstances or the manner in which the patients choose to respond.

Take Sally for example (not her real name). Sally appeared hyperexcitable, nervously talking and laughing simultaneously. Wanting something for her "nerves," she sought medication to help her calm down. Instead of improving, Sally's condition worsened, even harming her relationship with her husband. Seeking help from a Christian counselor, Sally revealed a series of life-events and her reactions. The counselor suspected the stress in her life had become so overwhelming

economic status. Someone born in poverty is less likely to be healthy and may have serious physical problems, especially in reaction to persistent stress.

Human beings' physical nature relates to one's biological and genetic makeup and what one does with the body. Engaging in healthy physical activity aids resistance to stress. Healthy diet and consistent exercise contribute to the body's ability to handle stressful situations. On the other hand, a lifetime of eating food full of fats, cholesterol, and sugar, combined with a sedentary lifestyle, produces an unhealthy body and, often, a sluggish mind. Similarly, work and sleep habits powerfully affect one's physical well-being.

An Integrated Approach to Understanding Stress

Not all stress is bad. Eustress (good stress) is vital to human well-being. People who lead someone to Christ sense tremendous elation. Their joy on a spiritual level produces a positive physical and emotional response. Long hours invested in reaching the person are like birth pangs, which are forgotten once the new babe in Christ is delivered (John 16:21). In a different scenario, some people need the motivation of deadlines to focus on certain tasks. While deadlines are stressful if time is not well-managed, the satisfaction of completed work can be almost euphoric.

The Biological Side of Stress

God designed our bodies to respond to life's emergencies. When encountering danger, adrenaline provides quick reflexes, pupils dilate to see clearer, and the heart rate increases, providing more blood to the brain and muscles. Hans Selye called this initial reaction the **Alarm stage**. During the alarm stage, when one encounters a stressful situation, the body produces substances that stimulate energy production and oxygen levels. They also affect the heart, brain, and muscles. On the short term, the stress reaction aids our ability to handle emergencies. However, if stress is chronic and intense, these reactions can negatively affect the body. Some substances secreted during stress have harmful effects on heart tissue.

Problems begin when the stress-causing situation, or our reaction to it, continues into the **Resistance stage**. The American Medical Association notes that as stress persists, people can be susceptible to physical and emotional difficulties.[4] Mayo Clinic physicians observe that sustained stress can suppress the immune system, increasing susceptibility to disease. It can also lead to asthma, gastrointestinal problems, chronic pain, arthritis, fibromyalgia, mental disorders, and other issues.[5]

If extreme stress, or uncontrolled reaction, continues, exhaustion (depression, illness, even death due to heart attack or stroke) can ensue. The idea of burnout identifies this tertiary **Exhaustion stage** of stress reaction. Symptoms include pessimism, a sense of meaninglessness, and feelings of hopelessness.[6] At this point, some people resort to suicide to escape their pain. Teens may engage in cutting, self-mutilation, or other self-destructive actions.

Where does stress come from? Stress can be endogenous or exogenous. Exogenous stress relates to circumstances external to the individual. Situations, events, and crises afflict everyone at various times. Externally caused stress can be relieved by dealing with the cause or adjusting to the changing situation. Endogenous stress may relate more to physiological problems (such as genetics or physical illness) or to mental and emotional difficulties. Evidence of endogenous stress includes unrealistic expectations, perfectionism, chronic worry, negative attitudes, and irresponsible behavior.[7] Endogenous stress may require medical assistance or the aid of a Christian counselor.

So what do we do about it? In this study, we will observe spiritual, mental, emotional, behavioral, and physical aspects of the human being as related to the causes, effects, and management methods of stress. As we have already mentioned, each aspect of human nature interacts with the others. Spiritual causes may have mental or emotional effects. Emotional causes may have physical effects. Physical causes may have mental or behavioral effects.

Sufferers may need a composite plan involving spiritual actions (including forgiving, trusting, loving, hoping), physical steps (like exercise, relaxation, diet, or medical help), emotional restructuring (such as gaining control of anger and replacing fear or worry with hope), mental reeducation (transforming the way one views life and solves problems as the Holy Spirit guides one into truth through Scripture), or behavioral habits (like deciding to act according to biblical, Spirit-directed ways instead of living in the flesh).

Not all stress is equal. The variety of human responses make measuring stress difficult. Just as people have different pain thresholds, even so they react to stress uniquely. Two people might encounter the same situation and one experiences distress while the other engages with eagerness. Moving to a new town might be an exciting adventure to some family members but stressful to others.

Consequently, **the issue is not the amount of stress but the amount of unmanaged stress one experiences.** Some people react to stressors more intensely than other people. Instead of taking challenges in stride, everything becomes a crisis, affecting them physically, emotionally, and spiritually.

Professor Richard Ecker, in his book *The Stress Myth*, argues that our perceptions of the situations, not the problems themselves, are sources of stress.[8] Some people react strongly to major life changes as if they were life and death crises. They can be so hampered emotionally they fail to engage properly in problem solving to deal with the changes. Others see the same experience as an opportunity for a new adventure. Conversely, while small annoyances are hardly noticed by some personality types, others react negatively to constant petty problems. Each person needs to understand how he or she responds to various types of situations and develop stress-resistant habits to manage each change successfully.

Factors Influencing Reaction to Stress

Spirituality

One's relationship with Christ is the most important factor in perceiving and reacting to stress. As discussed later in this work, people who experience the Spirit-filled life generally face stressful situations with more faith and hope than others. They respond to problems differently because spiritual resources provide inner capabilities for overcoming distressful events. The apostle Paul was able to be content with being either in difficult situations or in happy circumstances because of Christ Who strengthened him (Philippians 4:11–13).

Believers must choose to develop personal spirituality. If we neglect our walk with Christ and disregard our need for personal devotions, we are left to respond to problems in the frailty of the flesh. On the other hand, cultivating the Spirit-filled life enables believers to face challenges with the power of God.

Attitude

Stress-resistant people tend to have positive attitudes toward life. Their glass is half-full instead of half-empty. Their clouds have silver linings. Their world is controlled by a loving heavenly Father Who cares for them and is active in their lives. Some persons are naturally positive due to personality type, parental influence, environmental advantages, or other factors. Others have learned to cultivate attitudes of faith under the tutelage of Scripture, guided by the Holy Spirit, and encouraged by godly parents, friends, and other influences.

On the other hand, people whose first response to change is negative have a more difficult time with stress. They expect worst-case outcomes rather than believing God for better results. Perhaps they have suffered more difficulties or trauma in life than others. Pain tends to breed wariness of whatever threatens to inflict more pain. Other persons simply have assumed cynical, jaded attitudes toward life. They view the world around them as hostile and believe they must constantly protect themselves and their loved ones from harm. Instead of enjoying a life of faith, they suffer from various levels of fear that often hides just beneath the surface of their awareness before leaping forth when stressful circumstances inevitably appear.

Personality Type

Categories of Personalities

Personality types account for some variation of stress reaction. Typical categories include Type A or Type B behaviors. Type A persons are often driven, task oriented, and high energy. They tend to be demanding of themselves and others and easily fall into work-aholic lifestyles. Their encounters with other people can be brusque and may be viewed as arrogant and self-centered.

Type B personalities incline toward being easygoing and low-key. They often are people oriented and love group interaction, even taking a secondary role in relationships in order to find acceptance by others. They generally are patient, enduring, and quiet.

However, people are more complicated than these classifications. One cannot simply place oneself or others in a personality pigeonhole. Nor does personality alone determine stress interaction.

Another approach to personality typology is the DISC method, originally developed by William Marston and popularized through the work of John Geier. While understanding all people have some of each factor, the four letters describe distinct aspects of personality. D represents dominance. The D personality tends to be task oriented, proactive, aggressive, and bottom-line driven. The I (influencer) personality is outgoing and people oriented, wants to be liked, and cares more about social interaction than task accomplishment. The S (steady) personality loves low-key, easy-going, people-intensive group activity. This person dislikes sudden change, preferring the safety of familiar routine. The C (conscientious) personality is cautious, analytical, passively task oriented, and desirous of facts and order.

Responses to Stress

Each personality approaches stress differently. Some people enjoy a challenge and embrace change (as long as they initiate it) but get stressed by what they consider pettiness. Other personalities experience stress when their conclusions are challenged. A third group accepts change as an opportunity to meet new people. However, if the change involves conflict, some types become stressed. Perhaps the most stress-resistant personality is the naturally low-key, person who does not get overwrought easily. These individuals generally maintain strong support groups to help when challenges occur. At the same time, they react negatively to rejection and pressure.

Conflicting Interactions

The various personality types can have adverse reactions to each other in a family or work context. Driven personalities may view people-oriented personalities as shallow and perceive their need for social interaction as a waste of time. This person may see low-key personalities as lacking motivation. Dominant personalities can experience conflict with conscientious types who ask questions about procedures and accuracy of facts.

People-oriented personalities may consider dominant ones to be arrogant, inconsiderate, and bullying in nature. At the same time, they get along well with laid-back personalities because they like to talk, while the others enjoy listening. Quality-control personalities and people-oriented personalities can experience conflict because the latter likes to engage on a personal basis, while the former prefers remaining impersonal.

When persons with conflicting personality type interact, they will inflict stress on each other unless they recognize their need for one another. Each individual needs to realize that God made every person with traits that help other people be more complete. When all parties have godly love toward one another, various personality types become positive enhancements to personal growth and interpersonal engagement.

Thank God for Our Differences!

Understanding personality types not only helps us understand ourselves, it aids our perceptions of other people. Conflicts can be avoided and communication enhanced by applying knowledge of personality interactions. Relationships further improve when families, colleagues, or other groups understand each other's personality characteristics and appreciate their need for each other's distinctiveness.

Each type is valuable to the other types. Just as God gives members of the Church different spiritual gifts, which combine to fill all the needs of the Body, even so He brings people of various personality types together for each other's benefit.

Know Your Style

Each person's makeup involves a certain amount of each of these personality types. The combinations are numerous. Several testing instruments are available in print and online that can help you identify your particular personality profile. At the same time, one should be careful employing do-it-yourself analyses. Without proper training, misinterpretation and misapplication of results may do more harm than good.

Some instruments (such as the Taylor-Johnson Temperament Analysis) integrate personality and temperament qualities. Simple tests result in composite graphs demonstrating behaviors on scales between nine opposite traits, such as nervous versus composed, or depressive as opposed to light-hearted.[9] The Meyers-Briggs Personality Analysis is another test. However, each of these inventories tends to focus on secular psychological theories as opposed to scriptural foundations. While such instruments can be helpful to a degree, one should be wary of any approach that does not find its epistemology in the Word of God.

Temperament

A corollary aspect of human personality is **temperament**. Popularized by Tim LaHaye's *The Spirit-Controlled Temperament*, temperament typology focuses on emotional orientation. Choleric temperaments tend to be short tempered and demanding. Melancholic types often become introspective and worrisome. Phlegmatic persons may take life as it comes with subdued reactions to problems. Sanguine temperaments appear to be happy-go-lucky types who enjoy life. As with personality types, individuals have a mixture of temperaments and no person is solely one type or another.[10]

Related to stress reactions, persons with choleric temperaments tend to react to stressful situations aggressively, intending to overcome the problem by force of will. Melancholic types are often introspective, constantly brooding over problems (or perceived problems) with worried minds and fearful hearts. Sanguine individuals may seem to be the most stress-resistant temperament type since they appear to be energetic, happy, and engaging. However, their emotional expressions often cover hidden insecurities that flare under pressure, especially when they sense personal rejection. Phlegmatic persons range from relaxed to apathetic in their response to life. Some of these people may simply shrug off stressful challenges; others may appear self-controlled but actually experience inner turmoil that can have serious consequences if it goes unchecked.

On a more positive note, each temperament type has certain strengths in handling stress. The choleric individual may handle serious stress with greater assurance than other types. Phlegmatic persons rarely allow small stress to get under their skin, but see matters in level-headed perspective. Sanguine people engage life with a cheerful, optimistic attitude. While definitely challenged due to their tendency toward sadness, melancholic temperaments may have certain strengths in approaching problems thoughtfully and analytically.

The Bible offers many illustrative examples of personality and temperament types. Paul, for example, was strong willed, yet loving. He could be confrontational, but also conciliatory. He was able to reason intellectually, but was not dependent solely on rational arguments for belief and doctrine. Barnabus was an encourager of the brethren who looked for opportunities to lift up others. James remained strong in Jewish ethics and behavior, wanting to insure correct obedience to God's will while responding to the grace of Christ. Andrew, kind and approachable, was constantly encountering other people and bringing them to Jesus.

Whether considering personality or temperament types, we cannot simply excuse inappropriate behavior with the attitude of the comic character Popeye: "I am what I am and that's all that I am." God enables us to be and do more than our basic natures suggest. When filled with His Spirit, the fruit of the Spirit is freed to flow through believers' lives: love, joy, peace, patience, gentleness, goodness, faith, and self-control. Through His enablement, we can be better than we were and respond to stressful situations with overcoming faith and quiet hearts.

Learned Reactions

Another variable involves **learned reactions.** Through experience and education, people adapt their responses to stressors. Although their basic nature, upbringing, or culture may be disposed to certain reactions, they can adjust to manage stress effectively. For example, a person who has had a heart attack after a lifetime of poor diet, bad genetics, and hard-driving work habits can learn to eat better, manage time more effectively, and use new medications that can help with genetic issues such as bad cholesterol.

On the other hand, some people allow hurtful situations to shape their attitudes and actions into negative patterns, resulting in more serious stress formations. Growing up in dysfunctional, painful environments, some persons learn to overcome problems with aggression, while others may withdraw physically or emotionally. Constant infliction of pain can create scars that influence how one reacts to potentially harmful conditions.

We cannot blame our environment, experiences, or other people for how we respond to life challenges. However, by understanding how patterns of reaction have formed, we can be transformed through the Holy Spirit's renewal of our minds and hearts (Romans 12:2).

Gender

Increasingly, females suffer stress-related illnesses once thought to be unique to males. They have many demands, such as childcare and household responsibilities, associated with traditional roles. However, growing percentages of women follow career tracks with significant stress in the workplace, adding to levels of stress. Women tend to react to stress differently than men. Obviously, females vary between one another based on criteria other than gender, but women in general have certain commonalities.

Summary of Stress Variables

Each of these variables affects the degree to which people are able to manage stress. What may seem like a trivial matter to one person can be the proverbial straw that broke the camel's back for another. No single variable determines the degree of stress resilience people might have. Combinations of all the various factors are nearly infinite.

Of greatest importance, individuals' spiritual maturity affects reaction to any and all of these influences. By understanding our personal makeup and environment, we can more effectively cooperate with the Holy Spirit in handling components of life with grace, peace, and strength. As Paul said, "Grace be to you and peace from God the Father, and from our Lord Jesus Christ" (Galatians 1:3).

Chapter Three

WHERE DOES STRESS COME FROM?

Sources of Stress

Medical doctors use symptoms to trace origins of physical problems. Numbness in the hands can lead to a suspicion of carpel tunnel syndrome. Fever may indicate a bacterial infection or virus. Pain in the abdomen could indicate a number of issues related to internal organs. Symptoms tell the physician what tests need to be performed in order to identify the correct diagnosis. Only then can procedures or medication be prescribed to alleviate the condition.

Stress is different. A physical effect may have an emotional source. Emotional distress could emanate from a spiritual cause. People trying to manage stress in their lives or helping others dealing with stress-oriented problems must use observable evidence as warning signals. The flashing lights of stress' effects should provoke deeper analysis of the sufferer's life to find the source of the issue. Usually more than one problem emerges, requiring attention on several fronts.

Spiritual Causes

Sin

When God's people sin, His Spirit is grieved (Ephesians 4:30). The sinner not only senses the Spirit's disquiet but his own spirit is disturbed. God designed us so believers cannot enjoy sin. A believer who sins comes under conviction, which causes stress. Either the person repents and receives forgiveness or continues in sin with a hardening heart. At that point, God Himself becomes a source of stress because He reminds us of the sin. Sinning Christians tend to avoid Bible study, prayer, and worship services because anything that brings them into the presence of God is disturbing.

Bob seems especially touchy, Molly thought. He seemed unusually preoccupied and distant. Interactions with her and the children often devolved into bouts of anger that seemed to come out of nowhere. His work began to show signs of failure as his emotional imbalance bled over into the job. Matters continued to grow worse until Bob reached a personal crisis that led him to seek help. He finally admitted to having become infatuated with a woman who worked at his business. His illicit attraction produced significant guilt feelings that manifested in his attacks on his family and coworkers. Only when repentance and confession produced a sense of forgiveness and relief did Bob return to being the man Molly had married.

Doubt

Doubt is not merely an intellectual problem; it has emotional and spiritual origins. Stressful circumstances challenge one's faith. Christians are not exempt from wrestling bouts with doubt. Insufficient income, family illness, conflicts, and legal problems are only a few attacks on personal belief. When God seems not to answer their prayers, some believers struggle with their faith.

Doubt lingers like a stealthy enemy, denying its victim the contentment that comes from faith. People who harbor doubt often bear a distressed spirit as they wrestle with emotional challenges.

Anger

While anger is an emotional evidence of stress, it can also be a spiritual cause of stress. Anger is a natural emotion but often leads to bitterness and sin. Ephesians 4:26 indicates one can be angry but not sin. Consider the cause, expression, and results of anger. Human anger often results from the flesh or the self-nature (Ephesians 4:31; Galatians 5:19–21). While some people excuse anger as righteous indignation, rarely does our wrath proceed from a defense of God's character. It more often comes from hurt feelings, wounded pride, or personal frustration.

Human anger rarely demonstrates the nature of God (James 1:19–20). Certainly God's wrath is not sinful, but the rage of man and the will of God are generally mutually exclusive. Human anger often leads to sin, including bitterness, hatred, revenge, judgment, injury (Colossians 3:8). As a result, people need to learn how to control and cure anger.

Anger produces stress for everyone involved. Angry persons may express irritation as a result of stress afflicting their lives. The objects of their anger, as well as innocent bystanders, which often include family members, suffer the fallout of anger's verbal, behavioral, or emotional manifestations.

Correction

When we wander from His paths, God loves us enough to introduce correction into our lives. "My son, despise not the chastening of the LORD; neither be weary of his correction: For whom the LORD loves he corrects; even as a father the son in whom he delights" (Proverbs 3:11–12). We dislike being corrected and often resist whatever God uses to produce repentance. Instead of responding positively to God's discipline, we resist Him. Loving us, God will not relent as long as we remain in sin. The only real choice we have is to repent, confess, and return to our Father.

The process of correction, by its nature, causes stress. Internal disquiet of spirit presses upon us, moving us away from sin's attraction. In this case, the stress may appear as distress but is actually eustress (good stress) because its purpose involves our restoration and renewal.

Certainly, we could address other examples of spiritual causes of stress. You may be experiencing one right now. The solution in each case remains the same: come to Jesus. Don't delay. Remember the admonition of Hebrews: "Take heed, brethren, lest there be in any of you an evil heart of unbelief, in departing from the living God. But exhort one another daily, while it is called today; lest any of you be hardened through the deceitfulness of sin. For we are made partakers of Christ, if we hold the beginning of our confidence steadfast unto the end; While it is said, Today if you will hear his voice, harden not your hearts . . ." (Hebrews 3:12–15).

Physical Causes

Physical discipline, or the lack of it, affects how we respond to stress, and it can actually cause stress in other areas of life. Unlike the Gnostics of the early centuries who saw the body as evil and the spirit as good, Scripture teaches that we should care for our bodies as well as our souls. Paul prayed such for the people at Thessalonica: "And the very God of peace sanctify you wholly; and I pray God your whole spirit and soul and body be preserved blameless unto the coming of our Lord Jesus Christ" (1 Thessalonians 5:23).

To that end, the Bible encourages us to present our bodies a "living sacrifice, holy, acceptable unto God, which is your reasonable service" (Romans 12:1). Instead of surrendering to self-gratification, whether in sexual or gluttonous sin, we must discipline our bodies and bring them under subjection (1 Corinthians 9:27). Paul wanted to magnify Christ in his body, whether by life or death (Philippians 1:20). His prayer provides a worthy goal for each of us.

Some of the more obvious physical sources of stress include the following:

Fatigue

Weariness affects many areas of life. When we are tired, we make mistakes, use poor judgment, become angry more easily, and are more likely to compromise. Overwork, lack of sleep, long hours, and short nights tax the body and mind. When physical exertion goes beyond a certain point, exhaustion may set in. At that point, as someone has said, "The most spiritual thing we can do is take a nap." God gave His children the Sabbath as more than a one-day-a-week principle. He designed us to require regular rest so we can be refreshed and focus on Him. When we ignore God's pattern and push ourselves beyond normal endurance, we become more susceptible to stress in all areas of life.

Sometimes weariness comes as we serve God. Instead of pursuing God's call in the power of His Spirit, we delude ourselves into thinking it is all up to us. With good intentions and zealous spirit, we nevertheless substitute physical and mental activity for the fruit of the Spirit. When the body and mind finally start to shut down, we falsely attribute our exhaustion to the Lord's work and blame our burnout on Him. Paul reminded the Galatians: "And let us not be weary in well doing: for in due season we shall reap, if we faint not" (Galatians 6:9).

Weariness may be more emotional and spiritual than physical. David wrote: "I am weary with my groaning; all the night I make my bed to swim; I water my couch with my tears" (Psalm 6:6). His personal grief not only denied him sleep but drained him of joy and vigor.

God wants to empower us for engaging His calling within the power of His spirit. We can trust His promise: "He gives power to the faint; and to them that have no might he increases strength" (Isaiah 40:29).

Poor Nutrition

People under stress tend to eat comfort food high in fat and cholesterol. Instead of preparing healthy meals, overly extended workers grab quick and available snacks or fast food that often are counterproductive to good health. Substituting healthy nourishment for junk food, they do not get the nutrition needed for well-being, causing stress reactions to have a negatively enhanced effect. Too, fat and cholesterol can lead to coronary heart disease, stroke, and other physical problems. A high-fat diet also creates sluggishness. A high-fat content lunch may result in difficulty paying attention in afternoon meetings. Unhealthy people lack sufficient resistance to ward off viruses and other illnesses, adding to their stress.

While Christians are not subject to the dietary laws of the Old Testament, a diet guided by biblical principles will produce better health than the typical fare most people consume. We should take care of our bodies as the temple of the Holy Spirit. A healthy body enables believers to be more stress resilient.

Caffeine

Tea, coffee, soft drinks, and chocolate contain the Christian's "drug of choice": caffeine. Many people excuse their two- or three-cup-a-morning coffee habits as acceptable in order to provide needed energy for the day. Ironically, the caffeine addiction itself likely contributes to the morning sluggishness much like a hangover results from alcohol. Too much coffee can cause nervous jitters.

However, coffee is not the only source of the drug. Non-coffee users may revert to other sources to maintain their caffeine high. If you are a soft drink user, add up the number of ounces you consume in an average day. Take note of the amount of caffeine you ingest, along with the carbohydrate grams if the drink is not calorie-free. On the other hand, if you use diet drinks, do a study of the effects of aspartame before you start on that third diet drink of the day.

Chronic Pain

People who have not endured severe, chronic pain cannot understand the level of emotional stress sufferers experience. Pain from injury, illness, operations, and other causes feels the same—it hurts. Chronic pain leads some people to become addicted to pain-killing drugs, and it affects their mental and emotional equilibrium.

Ongoing pain, of whatever intensity, nags at the mind and body. Pain demands attention and causes lack of focus, often resulting in poor decisions. People with chronic pain may become less sensitive to other members of the family, friends, or coworkers. They tend to be more intolerant of whatever someone does or says that adds to their discomfort.

One of the most famous biblical examples of response to pain is Job. Although he stoically stayed steadfast through the initial losses, as time went by and his pain (physical and emotional) continued, he began to voice his complaint: "Therefore I will not refrain my mouth; I will speak in the anguish of my spirit; I will complain in the bitterness of my soul" (Job 7:11).

Paul experienced a "thorn in the flesh," which caused distress for several years. He prayed for relief, asking God to remove the problem. Most scholars believe Paul's issue was physical in nature. God declined to heal Paul, reminding the apostle that His strength was made perfect in Paul's weakness (2 Corinthians 12:9). Most of us would struggle with such a response. We need healing and we know the Great Physician is able to heal. Accepting His answer, especially when it means continuing pain, challenges our faith. It can make us or break us at the point not only of believing God but trusting that He can even use pain for our good (Romans 8:28).

Illness and Injury

Sickness and injuries create stress from the obvious physical implications and add to emotional distress. Family members find it difficult to watch loved ones suffer from ongoing pain. Especially when the patient is a child or teenager, parents experience pain alongside their children. They want to "make it better." Unfortunately, these kinds of problems cannot be healed simply with a mother's kiss.

One family suffered over two years of mental anguish as their child was treated for leukemia. The youngster endured scores of difficult treatments. He experienced remission for a while but continued to risk infection and other setbacks. He and his family suffered mental and emotional pain as they watched him. The toll on everyone was tremendous. Only through the grace of God were they able to endure.

Emotional Causes

Regrets

Too many people live in the "if only" of life. Focusing on the past, they cannot escape what might have been. Former sins and mistakes haunt their present and endanger their future. Relationships suffer when they drag the baggage of remorse wherever they go. Regrets include acts they wish they had not done, as well as opportunities missed along the way. They constantly obsess over small and large decisions that ended poorly. Just when they think they have left the past in the rearview mirror, the devil, that accuser of the brethren, beats them over the head with renewed regret.

God does not want His children living in defeat. Paul struggled with difficult circumstances and painful sins of his past, yet he found victory through Jesus Christ (Romans 7:19–25). God desires to set our sin as far from us as the east from the west (Psalm 103:12). Christ's blood cleanses the repentant believer from all sin (1 John 1:9). Through Him, we can forget what is behind and reach out to whatever God has before us (Philippians 3:13–14).

When we neglect such a great salvation and try to accomplish the Christian life within our own abilities, we inevitably fall short. The flesh is not designed for victorious Christian living. Without Christ's Spirit filling our hearts with hope for the future, we will remain bound by chains of the past like Marley's ghost in Dickens' *A Christmas Carol.*

Fear

Fear generally relates to some present consequence, circumstance, or person. Faith's opposite, fear can paralyze people, preventing them from making positive decisions that influence their future. Some people fear facing the consequences of past errors. Others believe circumstances of life always turn out in the worst way possible and live in fear of the future.

Paul reminded Timothy that "God has not given us the spirit of fear; but of power, and of love, and of a sound mind" (2 Timothy 1:7). The only fear we ought to have is the reverential fear of the Lord (Deuteronomy 17:19; Psalm 110:10). To the contrary, as we serve the Lord we can be strong and courageous, rebuking fear because God is faithful. As Moses told Joshua, "Be strong and of a good courage, fear not, nor be afraid of them: for the LORD thy God, he it is that doth go with thee; he will not fail thee, nor forsake thee" (Deuteronomy 31:6).

The great lessons of the Old Testament demonstrate how Israel mainly found itself in trouble when they were afraid of the wrong thing. Being frightened of their enemies instead of having a righteous fear of God, they made poor choices. Abraham feared for his life, so he lied about his relationship with Sarah to protect himself (Genesis 12, 20). Aaron compromised the entire nation when he made a golden idol out of fear of the people (Exodus 32). Israel wandered forty years in the wilderness instead of enjoying God's Promised Land because most of their advance team feared the Canaanite forces (Numbers 14:1–5; Deuteronomy 1:26–28).

The New Testament also points out the failure of fear. Nicodemus came to Jesus at night for fear of his peers (John 3). Joseph of Arimathea was a secret disciple until the crucifixion forced him to courageous deeds (John 19).The disciples were afraid of a storm (Matthew 8:26), the appearance of Jesus upon the water (Mark 6:50), and the arrival of armed guards to arrest Jesus (Matthew 26:56). Peter denied knowing Jesus out of fear (John 18). Pilate, although desiring to release Jesus, turned Him over to be crucified out of fear (John 19). The book of Hebrews describes people who were in bondage because of fear of death (Hebrews 2:15). Stress constantly accompanies the fearful.

We should respond to frightening circumstances by boldly saying "The Lord is my helper, and will not fear what man shall do unto me" (Hebrews 13:6). Let us not live timidly and miss God's glorious provision. As Shakespeare put it, "Cowards die many times before their deaths; the valiant never taste of death but once."[1]

Worry

Scripture constantly urges believers not to be anxious or worried about the future. People who lack a vital faith find themselves obsessed by what might happen. They worry over worst-case possibilities. Worry is the worm in the juiciest apple, the rot in the finest wood, the thief of joy and happiness in a believer's life.

Paul urged the Christians at Philippi to be worried about nothing, but instead to bring their requests to God through prayer and thanks-filled supplication. Such an act of faith produces the peace of God beyond our understanding, which will guard our hearts and minds through Christ (Philippians 4:6–7).

Mental Causes

Computer programmers have a common saying: "Garbage in, garbage out," meaning whatever you put into the computer is what you get out. Similarly, what goes into one's mind affects one's outlook. Paul urged the Philippian Christians to think on those things that are true, honest, just, pure, lovely, of good reputation, virtuous, and praiseworthy (Philippians 4:8). He told the Romans to be transformed by the renewing of their minds (Romans 12:2). We can fill our minds with healthy, godly thoughts or unhealthy, worldly thoughts.

The Desensitizing Effect of Secular Media

Christians rarely make a plunge into sin in one dramatic dive. Instead, they gradually become desensitized to sin by improperly using media that is controlled by people who dislike or disregard moral values. Watching television shows or movies that are violent, dark, sexual, profane, or are filled with secular worldviews will gradually affect any family.

Reading material that is not edifying can fashion a fleshly mindset. Believers should avoid those items containing pornographic or otherwise inappropriate content and stay away from materialism and other harmful materials. Magazines focusing on glamor and financial success lure readers away from what is edifying and good. Music and music videos also have a powerful impact, especially on teens.

In some regions, the nuclear family tended to be fairly cohesive and culturally consistent from generation to generation. Geographical limitations prevented cable television from reaching many of the homes. The satellite dish opened a Pandora's Box of sensuality for teens and adults alike, creating damaging input. The Internet multiplied the problem exponentially.

The Peril of the Internet

Internet pornography is a common source of sensual perversion and a growing danger among believers' families. Many people have become addicted to sexual content over the Internet. What once required a risky trip to the wrong side of the tracks is now available at the click of a button in the privacy of one's home. The advent of smartphones with instant Internet access adds a portable dimension to the temptation.

Unsupervised Internet access by teens and children endangers their developing minds. Curious by nature and fueled by newly discovered hormones, teens may experiment with harmful sites. Spamware pop-ups also lurk behind legitimate websites, waiting for naïve victims. Proverbs warns against the idle mind enticed by a seducing temptress. More dangerous are the virtual vamps who troll cyberspace seeking to pervert young minds.

the winter. Coping with daylight from 4:30 a.m. to midnight can create problems sleeping, creating biological challenges and resulting stress. Similarly, long periods of darkness have similar biological effects that can become depressive over an extended time. Sunlamps help in places with extended darkness. Hanging blackout curtains helps when daylight extends well past bedtime, but nothing ever quite overcomes the constant battle with light.

The above lists do not begin to exhaust the many causes of stress in our lives. As we have seen, stress is part of life and, as life varies from person to person, even so the causes of stress differ. What we can do is recognize the effects of unmanaged stress and take biblical, practical steps to deal with stressors in the power of the Holy Spirit.

Chapter Four

HOW CAN STRESS AFFECT MY LIFE?

Evidence of Unmanaged Stress

You cannot really measure stress, but you can observe the results of unmanaged stress. People handle potentially stressful situations differently. Their responses are based on a number of variables. When we say that someone is stressed out, we generally have seen evidence of unmanaged stress. To counter stressors of life in general, we need to recognize the symptoms.

Because different people react differently to life changes, one of the best ways to determine the levels of personal difficulty remains observation of evidence of unmanaged stress. If you experience more frequent and numerous effects, you likely have a higher degree of unmanaged stress. Problems generally occur not because a person undergoes stress but as a result of not reacting well to it. Consequently, as stress continues unabated and unmanaged, family, friends, and coworkers may notice a growing accumulation of various effects from each of the categories.

Psychological Evidence

Psychological effects may be the first observable signs of stress that has become too hard to handle. Levels of anxiety and worry appear unusually common. The person may demonstrate touchiness or ill temper toward friends and family members. A constant sense of sadness could surround the stressed-out believer, creating an attitude of always seeing the darker side of any situation and dampening any sense of joy or happiness. As stress continues unabated, some sufferers surrender to the lie that they are helpless to do anything about the problem, leaving them without hope.

Unmanaged stress can reveal itself in mental confusion, difficulty in concentration or decision making, and procrastination. Conflict presses so strongly that normal patterns of thought can be interrupted. Some people become forgetful.

Doubt and distrust also disclose changes in patterns of thinking, which can relate to unmanaged stress. As pressures build, some people start wondering whether God really cares. They question whether God is actually present and involved in their lives. Just as the disciples confronted Jesus as they struggled with a sinking boat, stressed persons might be tempted to doubt God and His goodness. Distrust also affects relationships with other people as sufferers project their pain onto persons around them.

When unmanaged stress continues over an extended period, reinforced by a sequence of hurtful events, individuals may take on a negative outlook on life. Instead of seeing possibilities, they only see problems. Instead of opportunities, they envision obstacles. One stressful situation may cause them to expect the worst-case result in all areas of life.

Emotionally, sufferers wrestle with anger, worry, fear, or regret. They swing between good moods and bad moods without evident cause. Little issues become blown out of proportion, injuring relationships— especially within the family. Overreactions do not necessarily result from specific incidents but from the accumulation of unmanaged stressors.

Children may complain of night terrors (nightmares). Such experiences often follow feeling threatened in some way, either in actuality or perception. Both conditions are equally frightening to a child. Parents should not dismiss these anxieties too quickly. Accepting the children's concern and helping them pray through their worries will help them confront and overcome the bad dreams and daily fears.

Behavioral Evidence

Accompanying the psychological effects are changes in behavior. Behavior reflects that component of human nature known as the will. Behaviors provide evidence of unmanaged stress. Some results-driven people may find themselves unable to relax, often refusing holidays or vacations and engaging in extreme multitasking. As stress mounts, they may begin to withdraw from associates, or even from their spouses.

Overeating or consuming the wrong foods can be one way stressed people compensate for their emotional discomfort. We often joke about stress causing us to eat comfort food. In reality, stressed people reach for their favorite junk food or whatever produces temporary relief from discomfort. Overeating is a pleasure without apparent moral penalty. However, as weight gain changes their appearance, some sufferers begin to lose self-respect and worry if their physique will make them less attractive to their spouse, creating additional anxiety and stress.

Other behavioral changes may be noticeable in personal and interpersonal ways. Persons who are normally well-groomed may begin to appear slovenly. Individuals who usually are open and friendly become reserved and withdrawn. Others appear uncooperative or aggressive. Habits and mannerisms may change either gradually or abruptly, sometimes producing destructive tendencies.

Some teens act out in inappropriate ways. Adolescents who have been stable, obedient children could begin to engage in harmful, even sinful, activities. More than mere hormonal changes, this behavior may relate to an overwhelming burden of issues they have not been able to resolve. Grades plummet as they have less interest in studies. Participation in extracurricular activities may fall off when they struggle to maintain emotional equilibrium. Becoming increasingly isolated, they either ignore close friends or reach out in inappropriate ways to receive peer approval and affection.

Children sometimes act out their stress at school or church. They may withdraw from friends and begin isolating themselves in their rooms. Some may extend their fears into their play activities. Unless parents recognize the symptoms and reach out to them, children's problems may escalate to unmanageable levels.

Physical Evidence

Effects on the body often occur as stress enters the resistance phase. The human body is amazingly resilient, but when it becomes overextended, unmanaged stress inevitably will affect one's physical well-being. Tension can produce constant headaches and other pain, sometimes resulting in the use of inordinate amounts of medication to manage the discomfort, creating additional problems. Physical effects also include problems with the circulatory system as blood pressure increases and the heart beats faster. Chest pain or angina may appear, in which case you should seek medical help immediately. (As a heart attack survivor, I know the importance of calling 911 right away!)

These natural responses to stressors develop into dangerous combinations when the alarm stage moves into an ongoing resistance phase, putting demands on the body that can result in stroke or heart attack. Many gastrointestinal problems can be traced to unmanaged stress, including indigestion, reflux, ulcers, constipation, and colitis. Physicians point to prolonged stress as an underlying contributor to many illnesses as a person's immune system comes under attack.

Ken's story is typical. He woke up one morning knowing something was wrong. The pain was different and greater than anything he had known. He had been experiencing intensely stressful situations over a prolonged time. Feeling unable to change the conditions of his circumstances, he had merely endured—trying to put a good face on matters, but inwardly experiencing churning emotions. Using inappropriate comfort foods, like double cheeseburgers, his weight had ballooned and, unknowingly, clogged a coronary artery. As the ambulance took him to the hospital, he did not immediately connect his failure to manage the stress with his present condition. He could only focus on surviving the pain.

Ken's story, unfortunately, merely presents one example of an all-too-familiar scenario. Overeating, lack of exercise, and unrelenting stress put a strain on bodies not intended for such abuse. If we forget our bodies are the temple of the Holy Spirit, we will suffer the consequences.

Spiritual Evidence

Believers also experience spiritual effects of unmanaged stress. A crisis of faith may ensue. Martin Lloyd-Jones' book, *Spiritual Depression*, describes spiritual problems that could fit into this category of spiritual evidence of unmanaged stress.[1] Spiritual effects of unmanaged stress may include the following:

Reduced Devotional Life

People who experience spiritual depression may abandon or reduce frequency of quiet times. Not having regular communion with Christ often leads to other issues. People who fail morally often spend little or no time with God in prayer and Bible study. Without regular nourishment from the Word and consistent communication with the Lord, believers lack the spiritual intake necessary for resisting temptation or managing life challenges.

Tom was a prime example of what can happen when believers abandon communion with Christ. Successful in many enterprises, Tom grew busier and busier. His travel schedule constantly took him away from home. Becoming stressed with the huge demands on his time, he ceased his regular devotional habits, believed he was too busy to pray. He also stopped studying the Bible. Weakened spiritually, he became involved in an immoral relationship. He lost his job and his family.

Immersion in Work

Most adults have a normal passion for their work. If they love what they do, they can find pleasure by spending increasing time on the job. Some people have a deeper drive to excel, either out of fear or from a desire to be the best in their field. They may begin to neglect their families and ignore their own physical and spiritual needs. Unless they break the trend, they might fall prey to burnout.

Feelings of Guilt or Shame

Genuine guilt results from breaking God's commandments, operating in the flesh rather than the Spirit. Shame naturally results from conviction of sin, just as Adam and Eve were afraid and ashamed after their sin. They had not been ashamed of their nakedness during their innocence, but knowledge of evil caused them to flee the face of God (Genesis 2:25, 3:10). Genuine guilt can only be relieved through repentance and confession of sin. When God forgives, we no longer are subject to guilt, fear, and shame (1 John 1:9).

Stress can cause believers to question their forgiveness. Experiencing ongoing problems, they may assume God has not forgiven them. Satan's accusation and an inclination to reflect constantly on failure can produce false guilt and shame. In this case, feelings of guilt have no specific object but remain vague and undefinable. Without specific sin to repent and confess, Christians have much more difficulty finding relief from false guilt and shame.

Lack of Purpose

Consistent stress often accompanies failure to accomplish goals. Many people weigh their worthiness by success and achievement. Stress can wear one down physically, emotionally, and spiritually, creating a weariness that results in a sense of spiritual wandering, without purpose or direction.

Feeling Worried or Afraid

Consistent worry or fear reveals one's attitude toward God. Instead of experiencing rest-producing faith in a God Who loves and cares for us, stressed persons exhibit persistent anxiety. They depend on self-effort instead of relying on a loving Father (Matthew 6:25–34). Consequently, they obsess with current and potential problems, unmet needs, and unresolved conflicts. In other cases, crises of life crash unexpectedly, driving normally peaceful people to the precipice of worry and fear.

Beth knew God loved her, but the uncertainties of her family's financial situation created constant pressure. Her husband, Frank, was immersed in his work. Focused on the demands of his business, he had thrust the responsibility of family management onto Beth. She was not prepared for the kinds of decisions she faced. Money was never abundant and, when the twins became ill, medical bills pushed their household budget over the edge. Financial and emotional stress took a toll on her relationship with her husband. Worry and fear nearly overwhelmed her until she shared her problems with her husband. He recognized his error and repented of causing his wife such pain and reassumed leadership in the family finances. Together they worked through the financial crises. Both of them learned to trust God to help manage the situation more effectively.

Faith does not erase the realities of financial difficulties or other problems. However, trust in a caring, capable Lord can empower Christians to endure when all efforts fail. God invites us to cast "all your care upon him; for he cares for you" (1 Peter 5:7).

Sensing God Is Far Away

Personal sin can result in feelings of separation from God and the loss of salvation's joy (Psalm 51:11–12). In such cases, the problem is not mere stress but sin, which requires repentance and forgiveness. Stress-related issues can cause believers to feel, without reason, that God has distanced Himself from them. Their prayers appear to go unanswered. Worship becomes formal and empty.

Serious, consistent stress can cause Christians to focus on circumstances and lose the awareness of God's presence. Although he was the king of Israel, David felt that way at times. When his enemies gloated over his difficulties, David prayed, "This You have seen, O LORD: keep not silence: O Lord, be not far from me" (Psalm 35:22). In truth, God had never left David. His troubles pressed upon him so heavily that it seemed God was silent and far away. I've felt like that at times, and probably you have as well. We need to remember God is still near and He speaks to us if we turn to Him in love and faith.

Having Difficulty Worshipping, Praying, or Reading the Bible

People do not cease having devotional times of prayer and Bible reading because they merely fall out of the habit. In reality, both activities have one result: they bring us into the presence of God. Both sin and stress can transform one's perception of God from peace-giver to stressor. We tend to avoid sources of stress, so we avoid God when His presence convicts us of sin or if we struggle to surrender to His will. Consequently, we fail to pray or study Scripture because we are uncomfortable with God.

> Unless we are willing to yield to Christ's direction, we will struggle with anything that creates an encounter with the Most High.

Spiritual weariness also creates disillusionment or discouragement that manifests itself in avoidance of spiritual devotions. While Paul urged believers not to become "weary in well-doing" (Galatians 6:9), the reality is even the most sincere believer becomes spiritually weary on occasion.

Ironically, the one place believers can find relief is the one place they do not go: to the Lord. He alone can give us strength for the task, determination for the fight, and peace for the spirit. Yet, unless we are willing to yield to Christ's direction, we will struggle with anything that creates an encounter with the Most High.

Difficulty Forgetting Mistakes

Everyone makes mistakes. Stressed people have difficulty forgetting them. The nature of continual stress makes people susceptible to preoccupation with the past. Healthy persons exhibit a level of resilience that allows them to move past the past. However, when stress builds up over time, they can lose the ability to handle mistakes. Regrets accumulate, creating a constant burden of reliving blunders. The devil loves playing videos of our past, filling our hearts with a sense of remorse and failure.

Billie Jean displayed a growing sense of sadness. Even when she and her family were experiencing what should have been happy times, she never seemed to enjoy it fully. She took care of her family diligently and was active in her ministry setting, yet her melancholy continued. Finally agreeing to talk to a Christian counselor, she reluctantly shared about a series of sinful actions that occurred earlier in her life. Remorse and self-loathing had robbed her of contentment and joy. These feelings had lain dormant for years, but a series of stressful situations brought them again to the surface. Through spiritual counseling and the loving support of her husband, Billie Jean finally found forgiveness from her past mistakes and began moving forward with her life.

Persistent Doubts

Shakespeare wrote: "Our doubts are traitors, and make us lose the good we oft might win, by fearing to attempt."[2] Questioning oneself, others, and even God may reveal more than lack of faith. Prolonged stress can make anyone second-guess everything and everyone. Lingering burdens weigh down one's spirit, wearying the sufferer. Resultant fatigue reduces resiliency when matters do not seem to improve.

We misunderstand the nature of doubt when we make it an intellectual exercise. Doubt is emotional in nature. Doubt and its first-cousin, defeat, afflict someone who is exhausted emotionally. Intellectual questions are rarely answered, for supposed solutions merely generate more queries. Sufferers may ask "Why?" as if understanding reasons for their dilemma would make them feel better.

Spiritual doubt may not be so much a crisis of faith as it could indicate an emotional reaction to ongoing pain. When unable to find relief from ongoing troubles, people may wonder about the nature of God and His providence. Like the disciples struggling in stormy seas, we ask "Don't You care?" (Mark 4:38). Jesus was able to calm the storm on the sea, and He is more than capable of calming the tempests in our hearts if we would trust Him and place our lives in His hands.

Excusing Misdeeds

Severe stress can display itself in spiritual callousness and insensitivity to personal responsibility. One of the greatest dangers for believers who sacrifice greatly for their faith involves a sense of entitlement. Having surrendered much in the service of the Lord, we can fall prey to the belief that life (or God) owes us something. If we accept this premise, we excuse misdeeds, discounting them in light of our larger sacrifice.

Maintaining Anger or Bitterness

Scripture warns that not handling anger quickly gives the devil "place" in our lives (Ephesians 4:27). Bitterness may reveal unmanaged stress because we are less open to forgiveness when we are under pressure, even if the source of stress has nothing to do with the source of the anger.

Tom was having numerous problems at home. Tension with his oldest son kept the stress level high. In an administrative meeting at work, a colleague made a comment that hurt Tom deeply. Normally, Tom would have been able to shrug off the pain or at least work with the teammate to resolve the issue. Instead, the underlying stress at home found an outlet in Tom's anger toward his coworker. Only when a third party intervened did Tom realize what was happening and took action to resolve issues at work and at home.

When Peter confronted Simon, the magician who sought to purchase power, the apostle recognized the man had been poisoned by bitterness (Acts 8:23). Paul warned the Ephesians about the dangers of bitterness, wrath, anger, and malice (Ephesians 4:31). A believer who refuses to deal with these sinful emotions and actions may suffer spiritual and emotional stress.

Disregarding Other People

People under stress tend to be self-focused. Even the most servant-hearted person becomes less able to invest in others while wrestling with personal pain. Members of one's church, coworkers, and relatives may feel slighted when the stressed person does not respond to them. Spouses and children often receive the brunt of the strain and perceive they are being left out of a vital part of their loved one's life. The offenders do not necessarily intend to shun others. They merely concentrate on their own problems so much that they simply do not see the needs of people around them.

Having Too Much or Too Little Regard for Material Things

Christians should not be materialistic—having a value system based on things. At the same time, believers have stewardship over whatever part of creation God has placed into their hands. People suffering from prolonged, unmanaged stress may exhibit two extreme responses. Some personalities go into a buying or accumulation mode, using the gaining of material possessions as a kind of comfort food to elevate their mood. Unable to cope with whatever is causing the real problem, they find their emotions improving when amassing more "stuff."

Other persons experiencing ongoing stress become almost oblivious of belongings. Completely focused on their burden, they fail to take care of homes, vehicles, clothes, or other material matters. Clutter accumulates in their houses or offices as they simply do not have the energy or concern to straighten up, dispose of trash, or take care of filing.

John's friends grew concerned when he became irregular at their weekly get-togethers and then dropped out altogether. They observed he seemed to be unconcerned about his personal appearance or needs of others around him. Visiting his home, they were alarmed to see the normally neat house had become dirty and disorderly. Sensing something deeper was happening, they intervened. Discovering a deep hurt he had experienced, they began helping him to cope. Once John came to grips with the underlying issue and renewed his relationship with Christ, he began to come around in all areas of his life and returned to productive interaction with family, friends, and ministry associates.

Evidence of unmanaged stress can surface in every aspect of our lives. Ignored problems rarely find resolution, they just get worse. God gives us many resources to handle life's difficulties. In the next chapter, we will find ways to manage the stress that threatens our well-being and endangers our effective service to the Lord.

Chapter Five

SO WHAT DO I DO ABOUT IT?

Methods for Managing Stress

We can't simply eliminate stress from life. While we might remove some causes of stress, other issues will inevitably arise. However, we can learn ways to avoid some stressors, reduce the effects of others, and manage those causes that we cannot eliminate. Doing so is not simple, but with Christ's help we can find ways to overcome these problems!

Remember, we are complex creatures. We have several integrated parts: physical, mental, emotional, behavioral, spiritual. Just as the causes and effects of stress can come from any or all of these areas of our lives, even so the methods for managing stress involve each part of life. Be aware that your unmanaged stress might be affecting your physical body but have an emotional cause. Methods for managing that stress, however, might involve spiritual techniques as well as emotional and physical ones. If the levels of stress are too great, you may need the help of a qualified Christian counselor to sort it out. Still, the following methods are offered to give you some ways you can begin gaining victory over the stress in your life and in your family.

Spiritual Methods for Managing Stress

God does not intend for His people merely to exist and subsist; He wants us to experience abundant life through His Son, Jesus (John 10:10). Christ alone provides what each of us needs, not only to manage stress but to be victorious over whatever robs us of the kind of life He came to give. While this book shares physical, mental, emotional, and other ways to deal with stress, without the work of Christ's Spirit we cannot begin to enter a victorious life. Jesus should be our first, not last, resort.

Enter the Spirit-Filled Life

Hudson Taylor called it the Exchanged Life. Watchman Nee called it the Normal Christian Life. Others have called it the Abundant Life or the Deeper Life. The primary way believers successfully live victoriously over sin, stress, and other problems is by entering the Spirit-filled life. Dr. Charles Solomon's counseling approach primarily guides patients to receive Christ as Savior and surrender to His Lordship in all areas of life.[1] As Bill Bright describes it, the Spirit-filled life begins when we confess our sin and place Jesus back on the throne of our lives. Yielding to Christ, we appropriate the fullness of the Spirit.[2]

Every believer receives the Holy Spirit at conversion. Paul wrote, "But ye are not in the flesh, but in the Spirit, if so be that the Spirit of God dwell in you. Now if any man has not the Spirit of Christ, he is none of His" (Romans 8:9). God's Spirit convicts us of sin, testifies of the Savior, regenerates the believer, and immerses the child of God into Christ (John 16:8, 15:26; Titus 3:5; 1 Corinthians 12:13). God wants us to experience more than just having the Spirit within our lives; He wants us to be filled with His Spirit.

With Christ at the center of life, we can be filled continuously with the Spirit (Ephesians 5:18). Living within the believer, the Spirit of God produces spiritual fruit—love, joy, peace, patience, kindness, goodness, faith, gentleness, self-control (Galatians 5:22). Stress cannot overcome someone who continually experiences the fruit of the indwelling Spirit of God.

The key to entering the Spirit-filled, Christ-controlled life is consecration, according to Hannah Whitehall Smith in her classic book *The Christian's Secret of a Happy Life*. Consecration is nothing less than abandonment to the Lord in all things.[3] Studies of leading Christians reveal how God brought them to a spiritual crisis in which they were forced to choose between continuing in the struggles of the flesh or surrendering completely to Christ. The Holy Spirit cannot fill us if we have not yielded every part of our lives to Him. Repentance of sin and receiving the Spirit's filling by faith also comprise the path to the continual filling of the Holy Spirit.

Hannah Smith calls this the "life hid with Christ in God." She adds, ". . . the Scriptures set before the believer in the Lord Jesus a life of abiding rest and of continual victory, which is far beyond the ordinary run of Christian experience. . . . We have presented to us a Savior able to save us from the power of our sins as really as He saves us from their guilt."[4]

Abide in Christ

We must be deliberate in maintaining our walk with Christ. Abiding in Christ means spending time with Him in prayer and Bible study. Taking time to enjoy His presence and commune with Him refreshes your soul and calms your spirit. Sometimes, your time with Christ involves getting by yourself. On other occasions, you benefit by having devotional sessions with your family or worshipping with your church.

Rediscover Prayer

In His most stress-filled hour, Jesus prayed. Before His arrest and crucifixion, He prayed (Matthew 26:36–44). On the cross, He prayed (Luke 23:33–34, 46). Jesus' habit of prayer gives believers a wonderful example to follow. Jesus prayed regularly. He often resorted to a solitary place to commune with the Father. "And in the morning, rising up a great while before day, he went out, and departed into a solitary place, and there prayed" (Mark 1:35). In the Sermon on the Mount, Jesus taught His disciples not to be worried about their daily needs, but to trust their heavenly Father and share their concerns with Him in prayer (Matthew 6:5–15, 25–34).

Unfortunately, prayer is one of the first spiritual acts to suffer when facing anxiety. Instead of going to the Father with our concerns, worries, and fears, we tend to withdraw from God as well as from people. Once we determine to reject a victim mentality and begin managing our stress, the first step is to reconnect with the Lord through prayer. If we want to trade anxiety for peace that passes all understanding, we must bring every concern to God in prayer and supplication, offering thanksgiving at the same time as an act of faith that God hears and responds (Philippians 4:6–7).

The Father loves to hear His children pray through the name of His Son. "Hitherto have you asked nothing in my name: ask, and you shall receive, that your joy may be full" (John 16:24). When we receive Christ, we are placed in Him and He comes to live within us through His Spirit. Praying in Jesus' name means more than adding a signature phrase to the end of our prayers. To pray in Christ's name involves reckoning our position in the Father's family through the Son and praying as He would. The substance and the spirit of prayer cease to be our own and meld with the intercession of the Son Himself.

As we revive our communion with the Father through prayer, we can share our deepest pain, our most fearsome anxieties, and our persistent doubts. He welcomes our honesty in prayer and responds with love and healing.

Repent

Regrets for wrongdoings drag believers into a morass of heartache and stress. Instead of wallowing in condemnation, we need to repent and confess our sin to the Lord Who is ready and willing to forgive us and cleanse us from all unrighteousness (1 John 1:9).

David understood that failure to repent condemned him to further despair: "When I kept silence, my bones waxed old through my roaring all the day long. For day and night Your hand was heavy upon me: my moisture is turned into the drought of summer. I acknowledged my sin unto you, and my iniquity have I not hid. I said, I will confess my transgressions unto the LORD; and You forgave the iniquity of my sin" (Psalm 32:3–5). Only when we turn from our sin and return to Christ can we find freedom through His forgiveness.

You may need to intervene and confront family members with their need for repentance and a renewed relationship with Christ. The apostle Paul took that approach with the church at Corinth. He wrote a strongly worded letter urging them to repent. They appear to have done so, because his second letter refers to the results of repentance: "For though I made you sorry with a letter, I do not repent, though I did repent: for I perceive that the same epistle hath made you sorry, though it were but for a season. Now I rejoice, not that you were made sorry, but that you sorrowed to repentance: for you were made sorry after a godly manner, that you might receive damage by us in nothing. For godly sorrow works repentance to salvation not to be repented of: but the sorrow of the world works death" (2 Corinthians 7:8–10).

Forgive and Accept Forgiveness

Receiving Christ's forgiveness removes one of the strongest sources of stress—sin. Forgiving others eliminates two other causes of stress: anger and bitterness. We do not forgive because others deserve it, but because God, for Christ's sake, has forgiven us (Ephesians 4:32). Jude prayed that God would multiply mercy, peace, and love in the people's lives (Jude 1:2). Few actions can relieve stress as does experiencing and expressing mercy toward others and oneself.

One man carried a long-time burden of anger toward people who hurt him as he grew up. Bitterness toward teachers, coaches, and his father hindered his effectiveness and brought him under constant conviction. Finally, he accepted the Holy Spirit's aid and completely surrendered his anger. One by one, he forgave each person. Having forgiven, he also had to accept God's forgiveness. The freedom he received afterward allowed him to experience the fullness of the Holy Spirit's empowerment.

Observe the Sabbath

Jesus said man was not made for the Sabbath, but rather the Sabbath was made for man. People need rest. God designed human bodies, minds, and spirits to need a day a week for rest and refreshment—spiritually and physically. Neglecting this principle prevents us from recovering after stressful activities and experiences.

Families should plan vacations, a weekly Sabbath, and regular rest and relaxation. We all need quality time for recuperation. Husbands and wives find their marriages and families strengthened as they step away from demanding schedules and focus on each other and their children. Children and teens also need time for recreation and interaction with their peers and families.

Combat Fear with Faith

Isaiah received a powerful encouragement during his ministry that has strong implications for believers today: "Fear not; for I am with you: be not dismayed; for I am your God: I will strengthen you; yes, I will help you; yea, I will uphold you with the right hand of My righteousness" (Isaiah 41:10). We can overcome fear when we remember the presence of God. He is always with us (Matthew 28:20). We need to remember Who is with us. He is our God. Think about that! The Creator of the universe is our Father and our God! We do not have a mindless, powerless idol, but a living, omnipotent Lord!

Isaiah also received the promise of God's power. The Lord strengthens us for our tasks, empowering His children with the indwelling Holy Spirit. When our strength slacks, He comes alongside us and helps us. At the end of our abilities, He lifts us up with His right hand of righteousness.

Faith is the opposite of fear and anxiety. Experiencing stressful emotions should motivate us to reexamine and reaffirm our faith in God. If we believe that He cares for us, we should be able to trust Him with our cares (1 Peter 5:7).

Faith Expressed in Prayer

Our first response to stressful situations should be to pray. Nothing puts us into clarifying communion with Christ as does prayer. Paul encouraged believers, "Be anxious for nothing, but in everything by prayer and supplication with thanksgiving let your requests be made known to God, and the peace that passes all understanding will guard your hearts and minds through Jesus Christ our Lord" (Philippians 4:6–7). Bringing our concerns to the Lord in prayer expresses faith that He hears us, that He cares for us, and that He is competent to deal with whatever we are facing.

Faith Expressed in Obedience

Andrew Murray reminded us that "obedience is born of faith and that faith enables us to obey God."[5] Obedience aids stress management by putting us into the center of God's will. We may not feel like obeying, but we obey anyway. Obedience verifies our faith. If we believe, we will submit to God's direction, trusting that He knows and wants what is best for us. Jesus said that our obedience demonstrates love for Him (John 14:15). Love and faith go hand in hand. Both are keys to overcoming the pressures of life.

Embrace Hope

Stress can be managed more effectively if people anticipate a positive outcome. Instead of allowing troubles to discourage and stress us, we can rejoice in the midst of difficult times. Paul wrote: ". . . we glory in tribulations also: knowing that tribulation work patience; and patience, experience; and experience, hope" (Romans 5:3–4).

We have hope because on our worst day Jesus is still Lord and our salvation is secure. We have hope because God is still sovereign and works all things for the good of those who love Him (Romans 8:28). We have hope because the Holy Spirit lives within God's children and empowers us to live abundantly. We have hope because we are more than conquerors through Him Who loves us (Romans 8:37).

Experience Love

Loving God, others, and even ourselves is the ultimate method for dealing with stress. Peace and love go hand in hand. "There is no fear in love; but perfect love casts out fear: because fear has torment. He that fears is not made perfect in love." Being able to love emanates from being loved. We are able to love God "because he first loved us" (1 John 4:18–19).

God also puts other people who love us into our lives. Each member of the family should share love with each other, their friends, and others. Sometimes, stressed individuals may not feel loved or loveable. Rejecting this lie of our enemy, believers should accept that God unconditionally loved us enough to his Son "to be the propitiation for our sins" (1 John 4:10). Living in His love, we can love and be loved.

Be Content with Where God Has Placed You

Many adults become displeased with their status in life and work. They may experience disappointment with results, disharmony with people, or distress over conditions. They may have thought they would have moved up the ladder of success, only seemingly to be forgotten. When tempted to be displeased with God and the location he has given us, we may well remember the story of Gregory the Illuminator.

Gregory was a third-century son of a politician in Armenia who became a Christian. The king, angry at Gregory and his father, put Gregory into a pit-like dungeon sunk into the ground, with only a small opening at the surface. Rain provided his only water. Each day an elderly woman dropped a bit of food through the opening. He lived for twelve years in his own filth. One day the king became sick. Unable to find a cure among the physicians and magicians, the king recalled the holy man in the pit. He had Gregory brought before him and asked Gregory to pray for his healing. Standing again above ground, Gregory chose to forgive the man who had put him into the pit. He prayed for the king. God heard the prayer and healed the potentate. In response, the king declared Gregory's God to be the one true God and his country, Armenia, to be a Christian nation.

If we knew God would accomplish His purpose through us, might we not be more content where God places us? The apostle Paul found himself in palaces and prisons. He knew abundance and abasement. Yet, he had learned "in whatsoever state I am, therein to be content." He could not do so on his own, but he could do "all things through Christ" (Philippians 4:11–13).

Fearlessly Engage in Spiritual Warfare

Spiritual warfare accompanies every believer's experience, but Christian families are especially subject to the attack of the evil one. The devil will use any means necessary to harm us. Only by a strong walk with the Lord can believers find the spiritual power to overcome our enemy. A vital part of spiritual preparation involves teaching all members of the family how to recognize and deal with spiritual assaults.

Parents must stand their ground in intercessory prayer for their children and teenagers. Praying for and with them on a regular basis provides a persistent appeal before the throne of heaven. It also models for the young people how they should pray for themselves and each other. Interceding for your children helps them understand just how much you love them. Too, hearing Mom and Dad pray for them with passionate resolve and confident faith gives teens and children a sense of confidence as they deal with whatever difficulties or temptations they might experience.

Mental Methods for Managing Stress

Acknowledge Christ's Power

Many secular approaches to stress management emphasize taking control of one's situation. Self-effort and mental gymnastics are useless without the aid of the Holy Spirit. Instead of merely claiming personal power during a crisis, we must acknowledge Christ's power over every situation.

Affirm each Scripture as it testifies to Christ's ability. He is an omnipotent God and has ultimate authority over every aspect of existence. Jesus has all power in heaven and earth (Matthew 28:18). Everything has been put under His feet, including those matters that threaten us (Ephesians 1:22; Hebrews 2:8).

Speaking helps solidify mental affirmation. Verbalize Scripture that proclaims God's superiority over whatever the problem may be. He is more than able to handle every challenge confronting us. He is able to save those who are tempted (Hebrews 2:18). He is able to keep us from falling (Jude 1:24). He is able to keep what we have committed to Him (2 Timothy 1:12). He is able to do exceedingly abundantly above all we could ask or think (Ephesians 3:20).

Reeducate Yourself to Think Biblically

How one thinks, as well as what one thinks, is vital to mental health and maintaining a positive spiritual attitude. We are called to be transformed by the renewing of our minds. One of the best ways to experience a transformed mind is to think about good and godly matters. Paul wrote: "Finally, brethren, whatsoever things are true, whatsoever things are honest, whatsoever things are just, whatsoever things are pure, whatsoever things are lovely, whatsoever things are of good report; if there be any virtue, and if there be any praise, think on these things" (Philippians 4:8).

Eliminate sources of temptation, whether television, movies, music, books, or Internet content that is ungodly. Place a filter on the computer's Internet programs to help family members avoid harmful websites. You will find it helpful to develop mutual accountability within the family and between family members and peers.

Learn to think biblically. When our beliefs and ways of approaching issues are based on Scripture, we behave differently—following biblical patterns of life.

Quietly Meditate on God's Word

Secular stress therapy emphasizes the value of meditation but lacks a spiritual basis. It usually defaults to eastern mysticism and yoga. Christians should reject the notion of using secular or mystical meditation. Instead, learn to meditate in a biblical way by focusing on God and His Word. While eastern meditation tells practitioners to empty their minds, the Bible instructs us to fill our minds with the Word of God. The psalmist wrote: "But his delight is in the law of the LORD; and in his law doth he meditate day and night. And he shall be like a tree planted by the rivers of water, that brings forth his fruit in his season; his leaf also shall not wither; and whatsoever he doeth shall prosper" (Psalm 1:2–3). By memorizing Scripture and focusing on God's Word, we internalize the thoughts of Christ.

Effective contemplation requires a degree of silence and solitude. Both are rare commodities. Jesus often left the disciples and went into an isolated place to pray (Luke 6:12). Spending all night in prayer with His Father was not unusual for Christ. When ministry demands became so constant that He and the disciples did not have enough time for a meal, Jesus called them to come away and rest for a while (Mark 6:31).

In a home with children, quiet times require discipline and creativity. Escaping the stressful distraction of noise may mean rising earlier than the rest of the family or staying up after others have gone to bed. Find a place and time where you can be alone with God. Open His Word and allow Him to speak to your heart as you commune with Him in prayer.

Focus Your Mind on the Lord

Whatever is the object of constant attention impacts our minds, pulling us toward that focus like a magnet. If we constantly think about money, or the lack of it, we become materialistic. If we obsess over our physical well-being, we can become hypochondriacs. Paul urged believers: "Set your affection on things above, not on things on the earth" (Colossians 3:2). The word translated "affection" literally means "to exercise the mind." The apostle knew the benefit of focusing his mind on eternal matters rather than the temporal issues of this world.

When our hearts and minds center on Christ, other issues slide down the ladder of importance. Instead of being captive to changing circumstances, our spiritual center frees us to think more clearly and biblically. We are able to approach problems with Spirit-directed rationality. Holding the things of this earth very loosely, we are liberated to follow Christ's leadership without the anchors of life dragging us down.

Embrace Contentment

Stress often arises when we lack contentment. We covet something we do not have. We want to be somewhere besides the place where we are. We desire a position beyond our reach, power beyond our abilities, or prestige beyond our talents. Instead of being grateful for God's wisdom in placing us where we are and giving us what we have, we become resentful that others have what we do not.

Paul learned to be content in whatever state he found himself (Philippians 4:13). Contentment does not mean to be satisfied with the status quo and not desire something better—for ourselves or our families. Contentment involves being at rest mentally, emotionally, and spiritually. Instead of experiencing angst or anger over circumstances beyond

> Contentment involves being at rest mentally, emotionally, and spiritually. Instead of experiencing angst or anger over circumstances beyond our control, we are able to receive whatever God places into our lives with grace and acceptance.

our control, we are able to receive whatever God places into our lives with grace and acceptance.

Paul passed his secret of contentment on to his protégé Timothy, advising him that "godliness with contentment is great gain. For we brought nothing into this world, and it is certain we can carry nothing out. And having food and raiment let us be therewith content" (1 Timothy 6:6–8). Timothy learned he could consider godliness and contentment a worthy objective in life.

Finally, Paul reminds us that we cannot accomplish this state of contentment through our own abilities. Our fleshly nature resists it. The forces of a worldly system conspire against it. Still, we can do this and all things through Christ Who strengthens us (Philippians 4:13).

Accentuate the Positive

Insomnia and worry are twin enemies. Generally, both result from focusing on problems—past, present, or future. Having a mind-set that gravitates toward the negative makes matters worse. Pessimists usually expect events to turn out poorly. They anticipate people will behave badly toward them. They are not surprised if life in general ends disappointingly. Negativity breeds stress. Pessimists not only suffer from bad experiences, but they also suffer from bad things that might happen.

Instead of dwelling on the negative, accentuate the positive. When confronting a problem, begin with the realization that your Father is Lord of all, including this problem. Believing the Lord is quite capable of dealing with whatever comes your way, you can trust Him and start anticipating a good outcome. Even if matters do not turn out as you wish, you will deal with the results with the strength and support of God.

Christians should follow the advice of that familiar hymn by Johnson Oatman:

"When upon life's billows you are tempest-tossed,
When you are discouraged, thinking all is lost,
Count your many blessings, name them one by one,
And it will surprise you what the Lord hath done." [6]

Developing a positive attitude does not mean adopting an idealistic, fantasy approach to genuinely difficult problems. We cannot simply put on rose-colored glasses to filter out painful realities. Instead, a positive mind-set involves choosing to trust God regardless of what may come. This way of thinking sees how God has worked in our lives and believes He can do it again. With His strength, we can tune our minds toward faith instead of doubt, courage instead of fear, and anticipation instead of regret.

Have Faith in God

Many people struggling with stress try to resolve difficulties in their own power. They rely on mental acuity, financial accumulations, human networks, or personal abilities to determine how they should live. While nothing is wrong with employing every available resource, our trust cannot reside in ourselves, but in the Lord.

Human understanding is limited by its very nature. We do not know what lies ahead. At best, we can rationalize, strategize, systematize, and organize. Yet, our stress levels remain constant because we cannot control the future.

Proverbs advises us: "Trust in the LORD with all your heart; and lean not unto your own understanding. In all your ways acknowledge Him, and He will direct your paths" (Proverbs 3:5–6). Instead of relying on human understanding, we totally place our trust in the Lord. The phrase "with all your heart" means completely, absolutely. This proverb promises that when we place our lives in God's hands, acknowledging Him in every aspect of life, then He will direct the way we should live.

Psalm 23 has a wonderfully comforting phrase: "He leads me in the paths of righteousness for His name's sake." When we totally trust Him and commit ourselves to unreserved obedience, God's name goes on the line. His reputation is at stake. So, we do not need to worry about whether or whither He leads. He will lead. He will lead in the right ways. His name guarantees it.

Cultivating faith in God affects our minds and emotions and has benefits for our physical well-being. Solomon reminded us that trusting God and refusing evil can produce healing and strength (Proverbs 3:8).

Emotional Methods for Managing Stress

People who develop habits of expressing positive emotions during stressful times tend to be more stress resistant and healthy. Obviously, people do better whenever they can employ humor, rest, or even recreation to divert negative reactions and seize healthy directions.

Focus Your Heart on God

Where is your heart? Not your blood-pumper. Where is the seat of your affections? What really matters to you? How have you established your personal value system? When our hearts focus on things of this world, we set ourselves up for stress. We spend our time and attention on matters over which we have limited control. At any point, whatever we love in this world can be taken away from us. Consequently, worry, fear, and other negative emotions run rampant through our hearts.

When our affections are focused on the things of God, we count material possessions only to be of such value as they can be used in His service. Having our treasure in heaven, we do not cling to the things of earth and are less stressed by their loss (Matthew 6:19–21). As Paul said, "They that are Christ's have crucified the flesh with the affections and lusts" (Galatians 5:24). Our emotions are liberated because they are pining for heaven, not pinned to the earth.

If we focus our hearts on God, emotions stabilize because they have a firm foundation. Paul prayed for the Thessalonians: "And (may) the Lord direct your hearts into the love of God, and into the patient waiting (steadfastness) for Christ" (2 Thessalonians 3:5). Love for God goes hand in hand with the steadfastness of Christ.

Cultivate Tranquility

Proverbs teaches us "A sound heart is the life of the flesh: but envy the rottenness of the bones" (Proverbs 14:30). The word translated *sound* refers not to physical health (although a physically healthy heart is a very good thing!) but carries the connotation of tranquility. How do we cultivate tranquility? By trusting Christ.

Personal peace comes ultimately from Jesus. He gives His followers a peace that is different from what can be found from worldly sources: "Peace I leave with you, my peace I give unto you: not as the world gives, give I unto you. Let not your heart be troubled, neither let it be afraid" (John 14:27). Temporary relief may be found from meditation or medication, but permanent peace proceeds only from the Prince of Peace.

Focus on Jesus and bring all your cares to Him. A tranquil mind and heart emerge from consistent communion with Christ. When stressful burdens seem ready to break through and destroy your peace, bring your concerns to Jesus, casting all your care on Him, knowing He cares for you (1 Peter 5:7).

Persistent prayer helps us keep our relationship with Jesus fresh and vital. Talk with Him about what is going on in your life as you would your best friend. Paul urged, "Be careful (anxious) for nothing; but in everything by prayer and supplication with thanksgiving let your requests be made known unto God. And the peace of God, which passes all understanding, shall keep your hearts and minds through Christ Jesus" (Philippians 4:6–7). Prayer is not merely a pipeline for divine blessings; it allows God's children to crawl up on His lap and cry, "Abba, Father," with all the trust and love such an act involves.

Interject Fun into Your Family's Schedule

"All work and no play makes Jack a dull boy," according to the old proverb. Scripture reminds us that "a merry heart does good like medicine . . ." (Proverbs 17:22). Whether engaging in a hobby, playing with the family, or simply appreciating the quiet company of good friends over a meal, finding godly ways to enjoy life is not sinful; it is necessary.

Children are not the only ones who need to have fun. The entire family needs personal and interactive opportunities for enjoyable interaction. We're familiar with the truth "The family that prays together stays together." They also need to play together. Activities do not have to be extravagant or expensive. Simple table games, hikes or picnics outdoors, or even an occasional game of chase around the house can bring a smile to the face and ease stress from the heart.

A young husband and father wrote, "One of my goals is to play golf or watch a movie once per month just because it helps me to relax a little more. My wife and I go on a date at least once every two weeks and that also helps a great deal in relating well to each other. I think for the kids, especially, it is vital for them to see their parents enjoying life and be thankful."

When unbelievers observe Christians, they should see a vital, healthy lifestyle. Enjoying life does not mean one degenerates into worldly frivolity, but neither does spirituality mean one goes around with a sad and serious countenance all the time. Finding ways simply to enjoy the life Christ has given us can help relieve tension and lift the spirits.

Learn to Laugh

"All the days of the afflicted are evil: but he that is of a merry heart hath a continual feast" (Proverbs 15:15). Approaching life with a good sense of humor helps ease tension and put matters into perspective. Spirituality does not require a somber countenance. To the contrary, the fruit of the Spirit includes joy! One does not have to become a stand-up comedian to combat stressful situations, but seeing the humorous side of life may provide the emotional relief to handle arduous challenges.

> Spirituality does not require a somber countenance. To the contrary, the fruit of the Spirit includes joy!

What others see in our faces generates from our hearts. Proverbs teaches, "A merry heart makes a cheerful countenance: but by sorrow of the heart the spirit is broken" (Proverbs 15:13). When children see parents' worried expressions, they worry as well. Conversely, when Mom and Dad habitually smile and laugh, the kids generally feel happy and secure. One does not have to hide genuine concern behind fake grins. Children, and especially teens, can spot a phony from a mile away. However, the normal tone of life in Christian homes ought to include plenty of joy, gladness, and merry-making.

Accept Your Acceptance

Many people feel rejected. I've interviewed adults who had lifelong problems because a father or mother only offered conditional acceptance as they were growing up—giving approval solely when they performed well. One young man wept as he recalled never feeling that he met his father's expectations. If he made an A on a test, his father questioned why he did not make an A+. If he won the silver medal at the school track meet, the look on his dad's face made it clear he should have won gold. As a result, he never felt accepted except when he excelled in everything he did. Unconditional love and acceptance does not mean avoiding encouragement to reach for excellence. Rather, it involves loving people just as they are, regardless of achievement.

Dr. Charles Solomon calls this the rejection syndrome. Solomon encourages believers to die to self and accept their position in Christ. Accept the fact that we are "accepted in the Beloved" (Ephesians 1:6). Being "in Christ," we do not have to worry about seeking approval from others because our Father gives us His unconditional love through His Son.[7]

When asked what was impacting his life in his later years, Dr. Dallas Demmit said he was "learning to live loved." Some people find it hard to accept love. Christians are quick to give love, but sometimes feel unworthy of receiving it. Living in the love of God and fellow believers is critical to a healthy approach to the Christian life.

Every member of the Christian family needs expressions of acceptance for one another. Parents must not assume their children know they love them. Children need to be told "I love you." (BTW . . . Kids, your parents need to hear those precious three words from you, too.) Wives need to hear sweet words of affirmation from their husbands, and vice versa.

Sometimes, you might do your best to demonstrate love and acceptance, but others have difficulty accepting your acceptance. Often, guilt for some past deed may prevent acceptance of love, or even of forgiveness. Emotional self-flagellation may be a poor attempt at making up for hidden sins. Shame strongly deters a sense of approval, leaving victims feeling unworthy of others' love.

We are not accepted because we have no guilt or shame in our past. Our acceptance is not conditioned on our actions. We are accepted "in the Beloved." When we trust Christ, repenting of sin and receiving Him as Savior, we are placed "in Christ" (Galatians 3:27). Our past slate is wiped clean and we are remade as new creations in Christ (2 Corinthians 5:17). Our acceptance does not depend on us but on Christ. If the Father accepts us on the merits of His Son, we should not insult Him by refusing to accept our acceptance.

Listen to Good Music

David's harp and hymns soothed Saul's troubled heart (1 Samuel 6:14–23). Even so, soothing and inspirational music can ease stressed emotions. Lyrics from good Christian songs encourage faith and hope. Worship-oriented music elevates the spirit, inviting listeners to focus on the Lord instead of troubles. Instrumental recordings can provide relaxing backgrounds, calming the emotions.

At the same time, music or any other emotional ointment does not heal the source of the stress. Dr. Jay Adams points out that Saul's relief was only temporary: "Saul's own attitudes and actions kept making his condition worse, as day by day he brooded with jealousy and resentment." Adams notes that Saul's problem was sin.[8] When sin is the root of stress, only repentance and forgiveness can provide long-term relief.

Sing

God inhabits the praise of His people (Psalm 22:3). We experience God's presence when our songs transform mournful expressions of grief into praise of the Most High God, our Deliverer. Joy comes in realizing His love, mercy, and grace. Stress melts away under the glow of praise sung to our Savior.

David, the "sweet singer of Israel," not only wrote scores of songs (known as the Psalms) but he obviously sang them. Many psalms must have been soulful ballads, written when David was hiding from his enemies. You can hear the pathos in his words as he offers his prayers to the Lord. Imagine David hiding in the cliff caves of eastern Israel, worried about his kingdom and angry over unjust attacks. His men likely listened in the night as he sang prayers of faith that later became the Psalms.

Christians can enhance family worship by singing praise to the Lord. Since each generation loves to sing songs of their youth, use a variety of songs. Children and teenagers like music familiar to their age groups. Older people may not know the newer songs, but each generation can join the other in praise through music.

As several families gathered at one home, worship began with a young adult leading the children in songs appropriate to their age. The leader then transitioned to music more familiar to the teens present. The final group of songs included a blend of standard hymns and contemporary praise choruses. Each person's eyes lit up as they sang, experiencing personal worship to the Lord.

Singing can often be best when one is alone. You do not have to have an audience or others singing along with you. Whether driving from place to place, walking along the way, or simply sitting at home, singing can change one's mood from sadness to gladness. As the Holy Spirit begins to fill your heart, you will begin to experience what Paul encouraged: "Speaking to yourselves in psalms and hymns and spiritual songs, singing and making melody in your heart to the Lord" (Ephesians 5:19).

Develop Stress-Resistant Attitudes

Some people seem to be more stress-resistant than others. They have as many stress-causing incidents in their lives, but they display remarkable resilience. Part of the reason lies in their ability to use good attitudes to shape their emotions, rather than allowing their emotions to rule their lives.

People wanting to increase their ability to overcome stress should intentionally groom their attitudes according to scriptural principles. For example, the apostle Paul saw God's hand behind everything that entered his life. Therefore, although he and his coworker Silas had been beaten and thrown into a dungeon, they were able to pray and sing praise to the Lord in the middle of the night (Acts 16:25). They may have been prisoners, but their hearts were not captive to their circumstances because their attitudes had been shaped by Christ.

Behavioral Methods for Managing Stress

Live with Integrity

When threatened on every side, King David relied on the mercy of God and claimed that he had maintained his integrity even in spite of wicked attacks (Psalm 26). Sometimes, people under stress are tempted to take shortcuts morally or ethically. In their weariness, they are susceptible to the lure of whatever makes them feel better. Maintaining integrity enables believers to receive God's healing. "Be not wise in your own eyes: fear the LORD, and depart from evil. It shall be health to your navel, and marrow to your bones" (Proverbs 3:7–8).

Since sin and duplicity lead directly to a stress-filled life, the best path toward peace follows the straight way of integrity. When you speak honestly and lovingly, you need not worry about what you said to whom. When you act properly and with good intention, you need not fear what someone might think. When you exercise integrity in each area of life, you can experience the tranquility of the upright in heart (Psalm 10:7).

Depend on God and Wait Patiently on Him

Sometimes the best thing to do is nothing. Yet, nothing is not always nothing. Waiting on God involves actively trusting Him to work in your life in His way and time. Instead of trying to take control of a stressful situation that appears beyond you, turn the circumstance over to the Lord. "He gives power to the faint; and to them that have no might he increases strength. Even the youths shall faint and be weary, and the young men shall utterly fall: But they that wait upon the LORD shall renew their strength; they shall mount up with wings as eagles; they shall run, and not be weary; and they shall walk, and not faint" (Isaiah 40:29–31).

Act

Stress tends to paralyze its victims. People experiencing prolonged stress may feel helpless to deal with their problems. Taking proactive steps toward ameliorating the situation produces positive emotions and hope. Jay Adams argues that behaving in a biblical manner affects our emotions in a positive way.[9] He refers to God's encounter with Cain who was depressed over the rejection of his offering. God responded, "If you do well, shall you not be accepted?" (Genesis 4:7)

Build Positive Relationships

Positive relationships not only help us manage stress but applying love reduces the sources of stress. Certainly we need to enjoy and strengthen friendships with people who care for us. However, Jesus taught: "Love your enemies, bless them that curse you, do good to them that hate you, and pray for them which despitefully use you, and persecute you; That ye may be the children of your Father which is in heaven" (Matthew 5:44–45). When we serve others, we may be surprised that our enemies become our friends!

Scripture constantly admonishes believers to interact with one another in positive ways. This list is not exhaustive, but imagine how much healthier and happier your life would be if you acted accordingly with your spouse, your children or parents, or other people:

- "Be kindly affectioned one to another with brotherly love; in honor preferring one another" (Romans 12: 10).
- "Be of the same mind one toward another . . ." (Romans 12:16).
- "Let us therefore follow after the things which make for peace, and things wherewith one may edify another" (Romans 14:19).
- "Wherefore receive one another, as Christ also received us to the glory of God" (Romans 15:7).
- "For, brethren, you have been called unto liberty; only use not liberty for an occasion to the flesh, but by love serve one another" (Galatians 5:13).
- "And be kind one to another, tenderhearted, forgiving one another, even as God for Christ's sake has forgiven you" (Ephesians 4:32).
- "Submitting yourselves one to another in the fear of God" (Ephesians 5:21).

- "Forbearing one another, and forgiving one another, if any man has a quarrel against any: even as Christ forgave you, so also do you" (Colossians 3:13).
- "Wherefore comfort yourselves together, and edify one another, even as also you do" (1 Thessalonians 5:11).

These admonitions and others can be summed up in Jesus' Word: "A new commandment I give unto you, that you love one another; as I have loved you, that you also love one another. By this shall all men know that you are my disciples, if you have love one to another" (John 13:34–35).

Manage Your Time

Master a two-letter word: NO. Some believers unnecessarily feel guilty if they do not accept every invitation, follow each opportunity, and fill their days with activity. In his book, *Margin*, Richard Swenson urged readers to build white space (uncommitted time) around their schedules.[10] Inevitably, crises occur. Without some margin of time, people quickly become overcommitted. Scripture reminds us that our days are few and precious, so we should use them wisely. "So teach us to number our days, that we may apply our hearts unto wisdom" (Psalm 90:12).

Work for Jesus

Interestingly, work can be an effective behavioral approach to managing stress. Certainly, many people experience stress due to employment situations and their reactions to it. However, work itself is part of life. Work can be blessing or bane depending on one's attitude. Labor involves more than mere employment. We work at home; we work at hobbies; we work at raising children. In every aspect of life, we work. The key is not working for ourselves, or even just for the employer, but for the Lord (Colossians 3:23).

Work was not part of the Curse related to the Fall in the Garden of Eden. Prior to Adam and Eve's sin, God said to them, "Be fruitful, and multiply, and replenish the earth, and subdue it: and have dominion over the fish of the sea, and over the fowl of the air, and over every living thing that moves upon the earth" (Genesis 1:28). Humankind was intended to be good stewards of God's creation. In fact, in creating, God worked: "And on the seventh day God ended his work which he had made; and he rested on the seventh day from all his work which he had made" (Genesis 2:2).

Sin's judgment caused toil to become difficult: ". . . cursed is the ground for your sake; in sorrow shall you eat of it all the days of your life; Thorns also and thistles shall it bring forth to you; and you shall eat the herb of the field; In the sweat of your face shall you eat bread, till you return unto the ground" (Genesis 3:17–19).

Scripture admonishes believers to be diligent in work. Using an agricultural example, Proverbs encourages us to be diligent in our work: "Be thou diligent to know the state of your flocks, and look well to your herds" (Proverbs 27:23). Illustrating from nature, Scripture goes on to urge responsible work while warning against the results of laziness: "Go to the ant, you sluggard; consider her ways, and be wise: Which having no guide, overseer, or ruler, provides her meat in the summer, and gathers her food in the harvest. How long will you sleep, O sluggard? When will you arise out of your sleep? Yet a little sleep, a little slumber, a little folding of the hands to sleep: So shall your poverty come as one that travails, and your want as an armed man" (Proverbs 6:6–11).

God's Word offers many principles and promises related to work. Joyfully engaging in productive work provides a positive approach to handling stress. When we do well in our work, our emotions rise, our finances generally improve, and we gain in self-respect. On the other hand, if we are lazy, we add to stress instead of relieving it. "He also that is slothful in his work is brother to him that is a great waster" (Proverbs 18:9).

Invest in Others

Stress often results as we focus on ourselves. Conversely, we reduce stress by committing our attention to helping others, being friends, meeting needs, or engaging in other activities that benefit someone other than ourselves. Seeing God bless another person through your effort produces powerful feelings of satisfaction. While being careful not to claim God's glory, we can experience inner joy as we watch people respond to His grace.

Everyone in the Christian family can find ways to help other people. Wives can encourage other women, offering words and works of encouragement. A fellow worker may need a listening ear. A neighbor could be stressed out with sick children. An elderly friend might be struggling with physical limitations. Every day presents some opportunity for us to serve someone else. Children and teens can also become involved in serving others. What greater way to nourish their appreciation for Christian service than to help someone else?

Find a Hobby/ Avocation/ Recreation

While relaxation for some people involves lying in a hammock or sitting back in the easy chair for a couple of hours, stress also can be lowered by engaging in enjoyable activities, such as a hobby. Through recreational activities families can enjoy one another and strengthen relationships. Stress evaporates as the family enjoys playing games around the dinner table, going on a weekend trip together, watching a sports event, or sharing a mutually interesting activity.

Be Faithful

Stress tempts sufferers to avoid their responsibilities. Physical and emotional weariness often become reasonable excuses for not making a meeting, helping someone in need, or following through with an assignment. Opportunities may be lost as stressed workers step back from their tasks. Ironically, instead of feeling less stress, people who succumb to this temptation often feel worse. They have merely added a sense of guilt and failure to their already heavy load.

> Be faithful to whatever task is at hand, even if you do not feel like doing so. Faithfulness produces a sense of satisfaction that often supersedes stress.

Be faithful to whatever task is at hand, even if you do not feel like doing so. Faithfulness produces a sense of satisfaction that often supersedes stress. Moses' leadership of a reluctant and rebellious people through desert wanderings caused him much grief, but he remained faithful. Doing what is right when things about you are going wrong produces a "Well done" from the Lord (Numbers 12:7).

Watch Your Mouth!

As you grew up, your mother may have warned you, "Watch your mouth." How we speak and how people speak to us affects our mental and emotional health. Words can even impact our physical well-being. "Pleasant words are as a honeycomb, sweet to the soul, and health to the bones" (Proverbs 16:24). We cannot control others' words or actions, but we can choose to speak kindly and graciously, maintaining personal tranquility. Scripture advises us to choose words carefully.

What we say can hurt or help others as well as ourselves. Gentle words can turn aside harsh wrath (Proverbs 15:1). Good words cheer the heart (Proverbs 12:25). Pure words are pleasant (Proverbs 15:26). Well-timed words produce joy (Proverbs 15:23). "A word fitly spoken is like apples of gold in pictures of silver" (Proverbs 25:11).

Physical Methods for Managing Stress

Relax

Taking it easy is not sinful! As we've mentioned before, Jesus told His disciples, "Come apart into a desert place, and rest a while: for there were many coming and going, and they had no leisure so much as to eat" (Mark 6:31). Having time to relax is important. Note the importance of having some time for leisure and unhurried meals.

Dr. Edmund Jacobson wrote that just as stress causes muscle tension, deep muscle relaxation can reduce tension and, with it, control reactions to stress.[11] Sit or lie down and close your eyes. While maintaining controlled breathing, focus on each major muscle group at a time, willing each muscle to relax. Completing the easing of the entire body, one remains in a relaxed state for a period of time, continuing to breathe fully. A few minutes of deliberate physical and mental relaxation can ease both body and mind.

Exercise

Physical activity is not only healthy but appropriate exercise releases hormones, which elevate positive feelings. Thirty minutes of walking or other aerobic exercise three or four times a week aids physical, mental, and emotional well-being.

Families can find ways to engage in physical activity together. Walking offers healthy benefits and an opportunity to explore the community. Children may enjoy skipping rope—an exercise that boxers also find beneficial. Teens may prefer more challenging sports, such as football or soccer. Badminton, volleyball, basketball, or other games also provide stress-relieving workouts.

Maintain Good Nutrition

Healthy living begins with solid nutrition that provides the body with the vitamins, minerals, protein, carbohydrates, and good fats it needs. People experiencing stress must be careful to plan, properly prepare, and enjoy healthy foods. While Christians are not bound by the dietary laws of the Old Testament, biblical guidelines for eating properly benefit good health.

A Few General Tips

Above All, Find satisfaction in Christ

Satisfaction in life should come in Christ alone. The stress and sin of dissatisfaction can trap believers who encounter persistent problems. Particularly at mid-life, some adults begin to evaluate their careers and wonder whether the outcomes have been worth the sacrifice. If they feel trapped in unsatisfying situations, they may begin to develop feelings of resentment and doubt.

One key to overcoming the snare of discontent is to find fulfillment not in where you are or what you are doing, but in the One you serve. The apostle Paul testified to his personal struggle with contentment and offered the singular path to serenity: "Not that I speak in respect of want: for I have learned, in whatsoever state I am, therewith to be content. I know both how to be abased, and I know how to abound: everywhere and in all things I am instructed both to be full and to be hungry, both to abound and to suffer need. I can do all things through Christ which strengthens me" (Philippians 4:11–13).

Maintain a Strong Support System

Support systems of friends, family, and colleagues are vital to maintaining health and overcoming stress. Often, simply having someone to talk with can help you unload the stress and solve problems. A strong support system also involves fellow church members. We all need others' prayers and encouragement. Occasional phone calls give the opportunity to talk about everyday issues and maintain relationships.

Grandparents can provide special support for children. Even if families live at a distance from their relatives, grandparents will find wonderful blessings by calling, texting, using social media, sending presents, hosting the grandchildren for vacations or weekends, and other activities.

Manage Conflict Effectively

One of the most stressful events in life is interpersonal conflict. Christians are not exempt from experiencing difficulties with other people. Not only do they encounter conflict in situations common to the human experience (marital or parenting conflicts, arguments with neighbors, disagreements in business dealings, etc.), they have unique circumstances that aggravate conflict. Time and space does not permit a full course in conflict management in this book. However, wise believers will study Scripture and take advantage of books and seminars to help gain skill in overcoming conflict.

The best way to manage stress generated by interpersonal conflict is to resolve the conflict. The chapter on conflict management (Chapter Eight) will give you biblical insight into understanding and resolving conflict.

Cure or Escape? Harmful Ways of Handling Stress

Stressed people often resort to methods of managing their pain that cause more harm than good. Instead of curing the cause, they try to escape the symptom. Inevitably, they sink deeper into the morass of emotional and spiritual struggle. Families seeking to manage stress must carefully avoid some of these pitfalls:

Alcohol

You may have heard someone who has had a bad day say, "I need a drink." Unfortunately, alcohol is often used by people trying to forget their problems. People who use alcohol to escape the stress of life end up having more stress. Consider Proverbs 23:29–35: "Who has woe? Who has sorrow? Who has contentions? Who has babbling? Who has wounds without cause? Who has redness of eyes? They that tarry long at the wine; they that go to seek mixed wine. Look not upon the wine when it is red, when it gives his color in the cup, when it moves itself aright. At the last it bites like a serpent, and stings like an adder. Your eyes shall behold strange women, and your heart shall utter perverse things. Yes, you shall be as he that lies down in the midst of the sea, or as he that lies upon the top of a mast. 'They have stricken me,' shall you say, 'and I was not sick; they have beaten me, and I felt it not: when shall I awake? I will seek it yet again.'"

God's litany of wisdom includes warnings against the dangers of alcohol:

- "Wine is a mocker, strong drink is raging: and whosoever is deceived thereby is not wise" (Proverbs 20:1).
- "It is not for kings, O Lemuel, it is not for kings to drink wine; nor for princes strong drink: Lest they drink, and forget the law, and pervert the judgment of any of the afflicted" (Proverbs 31:4–5).
- "Woe unto them that are mighty to drink wine, and men of strength to mingle strong drink: Which justify the wicked for reward, and take away the righteousness of the righteous from him!" (Isaiah 5:22–23).
- "Woe unto them that rise up early in the morning, that they may follow strong drink; that continue until night, till wine inflame them!" (Isaiah 5:11).
- "But they also have erred through wine, and through strong drink are out of the way; the priest and the prophet have

erred through strong drink, they are swallowed up of wine, they are out of the way through strong drink; they err in vision, they stumble in judgment" (Isaiah 28:7).

Hannah was a woman who experienced extreme stress. She was childless and wanted a baby desperately. She could have responded to her situation in many ways, but listen to her testimony: "I am a woman of a sorrowful spirit: I have drunk neither wine nor strong drink, but have poured out my soul before the LORD" (1 Samuel 1:15). Instead of drowning her sorrows in liquor, she brought her problem to God!

Most believers experience no attraction to alcohol. Their Christian commitment keeps them from using substances that hurt their witness and harm their prospects of winning the people to Jesus. At the same time, particularly if individuals had a history of alcohol use before salvation, the temptation to drown one's sorrows remains a real challenge.

Drugs

Some people use drugs to alter their moods. Marijuana, cocaine, ecstasy, and other drugs are designed to produce euphoric feelings, but, in the end, have disastrous results physically, emotionally, and spiritually. Amphetamines raise a person's alertness, but become highly addictive, alter one's moods, and can produce hallucinations. Amphetamines have been linked to heart attacks, strokes, and other causes of sudden death. Barbiturates are often used for sedation or anxiety, but also produce sluggishness, poor judgment, and even death.

Few Christians resort to these drugs but may be tempted to abuse prescription pharmaceuticals, including pain killers, sleep aids, and diet pills (which often contain substances with amphetamine-like properties). Medications meant to elevate depressed persons can become substitutes for dealing with the spiritual issues behind the sorrowful moods.

Sex

God created sex as a beautiful part of human life. Not only designed for procreation, sex was intended to express ultimate intimacy between a husband and wife. Emotional benefits likely outrank physical pleasure among the blessings of a loving sexual relationship. Scripture offers wise advice about the marriage covenant: ". . . rejoice with the wife of thy youth. Let her be as the loving hind and pleasant roe; let her breasts satisfy you at all times; and be ravished always with her love" (Proverbs 5:15–19).

Unfortunately, some people abuse sex. When a woman senses her husband wants to have sex simply to relieve stress, she feels used. Instead of feeling affirmation and love, she becomes an object for another's selfish satisfaction. Rightly employed in a mutually giving act of love between a husband and wife, sex builds marriages up. Wrongly exploited for self-gratification, it quickly tears down years of trust and tenderness. Sexual intimacy should be the most fulfilling expression of love and oneness in a marriage. It should not be reduced to a stress-management technique.

Shopping

Some people go on spending sprees when under stress. If spending money becomes a temporary antidote for dissatisfaction, discouragement, or depression, it ceases being productive and often adds financial burdens to an already stressful environment. This problem is not limited to females. Men also misuse money during stress; only their purchases can be more costly and, in the case of escapism, more detrimental.

Escapism

Under stress, people look for an escape or, at least, a distraction. They often withdraw from relationships or interaction with family and friends. Instead of recognizing the source of the stress and dealing with it honestly and openly, they become vulnerable to temptations that promise a break.

The Internet has become one of the most common and dangerous vehicles for escape. While the Net provides a wonderful way for the family to get information, conduct business, and maintain communication with distant friends and family, many Christian families have been torn apart by inappropriate and sinful misuse.

Christian families are not immune from becoming involved with unknown persons in an online chat room. Pornography also sits in cyberspace like a coiled adder, waiting to strike foolish folk who fool around with its hidden lures. Thinking no one will know, men and women (as well as teens, and even some children) regularly enter a world of fantasy and lust. They ignore godly wisdom: "Stolen waters are sweet, and bread eaten in secret is pleasant. But he knows not that the dead are there; and that her guests are in the depths of hell" (Proverbs 9:17–18).

Some people find themselves addicted to sexual perversions. Left unchecked, their licentious appetites demand increasingly more lurid fantasies. All sorts of sexual sins lie at their door waiting to destroy them. Scripture warns: "When wisdom enters into your heart, and knowledge is pleasant unto your soul; Discretion shall preserve you, understanding shall keep you To deliver you from the way of the evil man, . . . Whose ways are crooked, . . . To deliver you from the strange woman, even from the stranger which flatters with her words; Which forsakes the guide of her youth, and forgets the covenant of her God, for her house inclines unto death, and her paths unto the dead" (Proverbs 2:10–18).

Christians caught in the Internet porn trap find themselves broken when caught by their spouse, or, worse, their children. Many marriages have ended, with children, churches, family, and friends left in the wreckage. Through much counseling, sorrow, and repentance, they may receive forgiveness and reconciliation.

Chapter Six

WHAT ELSE CAN I DO TO HELP MY MARRIAGE AND FAMILY?

Marriage and Family Issues

One of the first lines of defense against overwhelming stress is a godly home. Just as the home is one of the basic building blocks of society, even so the family is a central component of ministry. The Christian home is a secure place where family members nurture one another, and the haven to which they can resort at the end of stressful days. Sustaining strong marriages and healthy families should be a top priority. The dynamics of life in a postmodern context make these goals more difficult to attain and, at the same time, more important to maintain. The starting place commences with developing strong marriages.

Strengthening Marital Relationships

If parents want to provide a healthy environment for their children, they must relate well with one another. Many marriage counselors refer to Ephesians 5 when describing the qualities of a successful marriage. The godly husband loves the wife and gives himself to her sacrificially. The spiritual spouse submits to her husband as unto the Lord, trusting God to guide him as the spiritual leader of the home. The two mutually serve one another in Christian love. While these truths are vital, they are only two aspects of healthy relationships.

Base Your Commitment to Each Other on Your Commitment to Christ

"Except the LORD build the house, they labor in vain that build it: . ." (Psalm 127:1). In marriage counseling, I don't put the first emphasis on discovering the couple's problems. Instead, we focus on each person's relationship with Christ. If both people draw closer to Jesus, they will naturally come nearer one another. A successful, happy marriage begins with a husband and wife who love Jesus and live with Him as Lord.

Pray for one another and encourage each other in your relationships with Jesus. Reading the Scriptures and worshipping together will strengthen your mutual bond with the Lord and with one another. The more you love Christ, the stronger your affection will be for each other. In addition, your expression of devotion to Jesus and care for one another will provide a strong model for your children.

Treat One Another as You Want to Be Treated

Jesus' admonition to do unto others as we would want them to do unto us should be employed in the home before it can occur elsewhere (Matthew 7:12). The New Testament's "one anothering" passages, mentioned earlier in this work, apply not only to relationships within the church, but they have special application to husbands and wives. Marriages grow stronger as husbands and wives exercise commitments such as these to one another:

- **Encourage one another to love and good works.** (Hebrews 10:24) Loving families find ways to encourage one another in general, specifically to "love and good works." Helping each other express love in practical ways blesses the other person and provides a solid basis for mutual satisfaction.
- **Comfort and edify one another.** (1 Thessalonians 5:11) Everyone gets down at times. Whenever a husband or wife experiences sadness, the spouse need not try immediately to fix the problem, but should simply offer comfort and encouragement. Genuine empathy is one way to comfort

one another. The Bible advises us to laugh with those who laugh and weep with those who weep (Romans 12:15).

- **Speak well to one another.** (Colossians 3:8–9) One never builds a marriage up by putting the other person down. How we speak to one another can edify and encourage or cause deep pain. Couples must guard their communication. Avoid speaking in anger. Don't lie to one another. Instead, use words to share feelings honestly without attacking the other person. Intending to help one another, we will choose words that help and not hurt.

- **Lovingly serve one another.** (Galatians 5:13) Wedding vows often include the phrase "Do you promise to love, honor, trust, and serve one another in sickness and in health, in adversity and prosperity, and to be true and faithful to one another as long as you both shall live?" True love finds ways to serve the one who is loved. Husbands, don't wait until you are asked to help with the dishes; just pick up a cloth and start washing! Wives can also find ways to serve their husbands with more than just a meal.

- **Be kind and affectionate toward one another.** (Romans 12:10) Kindness makes deposits in relational accounts that sustain families during times of tension and stress. Genuine affection expresses itself in hugs and kisses, as well as kind words and deeds.

- **Confess your faults and pray for one another.** (James 5:16) Instead of hiding or excusing errors, confess mistakes to one another. When one spouse offers honest, contrite confession, the receiving spouse responds with acceptance and forgiveness. Praying for each other is a powerful tool for building strong relationships.

- **Grudge not one against another.** (James 5:9) One test of genuine forgiveness involves whether a past sin comes back up in future arguments. Godly love does not bear grudges (1 Corinthians 13:5).

- **Forbear and forgive one another.** (Colossians 3:13) The idea of forbearance involves restraint. When injured, our natural inclination is to lash out in anger and retaliation.

Many marital struggles begin with reaction to pain. Paul's advice is to restrain oneself and forgive the other person. If we remember how Christ has forgiven us, we can find motivation to forgive others.

> Godly love does not bear grudges.

Appreciate the Differences in Your Personalities

Opposites attract, so the old saying goes. Often men and women with very different personalities marry. Sometimes they become frustrated with one another, often because they do not understand how each completes the other. When we first married, my wife and I had numerous occasions where our differing personalities clashed. Once we learned how our personality types complemented one another, we began to appreciate how God put us together so each one's strengths made up for the other's weaknesses.

Maintain Communication

During tension and stress, one of the first victims is communication. Men tend not to be communicative even on a good day. Small talk is not our strong point. Under pressure, we clam up even more. "How's your day, honey?" the wife might ask. "Okay," grunts the husband. Wives may understand that their husbands are under stress, but they perceive the lack of communication as if their spouses are shutting them out.

Whether stress originates within the marriage or emerges from other causes, committed couples cannot yield to the temptation to withdraw emotionally. If tension has resulted from a perceived offense, a misspoken word or hurtful action, husbands and wives must talk through the issue to a resolution. Down-playing or discounting the pain does not help. Simply saying, "Never mind, it's nothing," solves nothing. Maintaining honest and kind communication helps solve problems, encourages others, and deepens relationships.

Keep the Flame of Love Alive

Wise husbands look for opportunities to rekindle romance. While serving in state missions, I traveled fifty thousand miles a year in my car and had to spend two hundred nights each year in hotels. When I finally arrived home on Friday night, the last thing I wanted to do was get back in the car and go out for yet another meal that was not home cooked. Realizing my wife had been taking care of the children all week and working her own job as a piano teacher, I discovered ways to enhance our relationship. In our case, we spent Friday night at home as a family. We called it "Friday Family Fun Night," interjecting a good home-cooked meal with fun activities the entire family enjoyed. Then, on Saturday night, my wife and I usually had a date night. Without having to invest a small fortune in fancy restaurants or expensive places, we found many ways to revisit our courtship. Each date was a reinvestment in our relationship. After forty-five years of marriage, we still make date nights an important part of our lifestyle.

Wives also have responsibilities to make romance work amidst hectic schedules. Families with children can sometimes trade off nights of childcare, giving each couple some time alone. Candlelight dinners at home may be just as romantic as an expensive night at a four-star restaurant.

Husbands and wives should take care of their appearances. Men should realize that work, especially outdoors or in an environment without air conditioning, means they need to bathe and shave before reaching for a hug and a kiss. The pleasure of renewed romance is worth the effort.

Enjoy Intimacy

Sex is much more than a physical act. It should express the deepest emotional intimacy a husband and wife can experience. Among the demands of children, work, travel, and other aspects of life, couples may become stressed by the lack of private time together.

Husbands and wives may express frustration from inadequate emotional connection and affirmation in their marital relationship.

111

Couples should make a priority of maintaining a high level of personal intimacy, emotionally and physically. As Paul said: "Let the husband render unto the wife due benevolence: and likewise also the wife unto the husband. . . . Defraud ye not one the other, except it be with consent for a time, that ye may give yourselves to fasting and prayer; and come together again, that Satan tempt you not for your incontinency" (1 Corinthians 7:3–5).

Resolve Conflict Quickly and Quietly

Every couple experiences disagreements. Unfortunately, some disagreements degenerate into conflict. The chapter on conflict management (Chapter Eight) shares many principles that can be used in resolving marital disharmony. Here, let us focus on two key issues for resolving marriage conflict.

First, resolve struggles quickly. "Don't let the sun go down on your wrath" (Ephesians 4:26). Delaying solutions often makes matters worse. As I prepared for marriage, my mother advised, "Son, never go to bed mad." She was right. Settle disputes quickly. When problems fester like an untreated sore, they can damage relationships.

Second, handle disagreements quietly. Some people grow up in homes where parents raised their voices while arguing. Others had homes characterized by peace and parents who worked out their problems without shouting. People often repeat the models of their childhood, bringing unhealthy patterns of coping into their marriages. Loud arguments rarely end well. "A soft answer turns aside wrath" (Proverbs 15:1).

Children become fearful when their parents' argue. If conflict continues or degenerates into shouting matches, children can be traumatized. They may begin having night terrors if they sense their security is threatened. On the other hand, some children may act out their anger toward other children, siblings, or even the parents. Quick and quiet conflict resolution models a healthy approach for children and helps build stronger marriages.

With unconditional love for each other and total commitment to their marriage, husbands and wives can find ways to improve their relationships. Christian couples can access numerous Christian books and other resources to give them additional insights into keeping their marriages strong. Biblical counseling can help couples with severe difficulties resolve their differences. Their greatest aid is the Holy Spirit Who works within each of them to meld the two into one.

Raising Godly Children

"Lo, children are a heritage of the LORD: and the fruit of the womb is his reward" (Psalm 127:3). Couples blessed with children understand the duality of pleasure and pain child-rearing can be. Nurturing children is challenging, but it provides a wonderful opportunity for both parents and children. This small section cannot address all the issues of child-rearing, but it includes four areas that tend to be especially stressful: childbearing, education, discipline, and dealing with prodigals.

Childbearing

Husbands cannot fully comprehend the dynamics a woman experiences during nine months of pregnancy and hours of painful childbirth. We can, however, be supportive and understanding. Wives can help their clueless husbands by sharing what's happening to them physically and emotionally. As the couple works through the blessed event together, they can find their relationship growing deeper.

Building a support network in anticipation of childbirth can reduce the stress. Existing children may need someone to care for them while the parents are busy with the birth. If a couple does not have the advantage of having extended family nearby, mothers-to-be rely more heavily on friends and physicians. Sometimes, the extended family, especially the woman's mother, may be able to stay with the couple for a while to help out with other children, housework, cooking, and general encouragement. If she does, she needs to understand her role is supportive; she must resist the temptation to take over her daughter's household.

Providing Education

Educating children and teens can be a challenge. Many choices are available, but each has its own stress. The public education system offers many advantages, but in some places the environment or the values of the system may not be conducive to raising Christian kids. Some parents may choose private, usually church-related, schools.

Some parents choose to homeschool their children, particularly those in elementary school, although increasingly more high-school students are successfully homeschooled. The advantages include control over curriculum, convenience, costs, schedule flexibility, and security. Disadvantages can be stressful. Children may have difficulty separating the roles of the parent tasked with teaching (usually the mother). When are you the mom and when are you the teacher? When a child does not do well in schoolwork or becomes unruly, who exercises discipline: the mother or the teacher? Too, the teacher/parent never has a break from interaction with the children, often producing exhaustive stress.

One answer involves several families creating a homeschool cooperative, in which parents share in various responsibilities. While problems can be overcome, the entire family has to work with one another to produce a happy solution.

Discipline and Discipling

Correction not only is necessary but is an act of love. If a child or teenager misbehaves in attitude or action, only an unloving parent would ignore or excuse the problem. To allow disobedience to go on undisciplined encourages the child to continue down a destructive path. Scripture reminds us that just as a parent lovingly disciplines children, even so the heavenly Father corrects those He loves (Hebrews 12:6–7).

Discipline in typical families falls to the father. In some homes, particularly if Dad has to travel for a living, the mother must assume the responsibility for correction. Regardless of which parent executes discipline, the manner in which children are corrected is important. Paul warned that punishment should not be so harsh that children lose heart and rebel. "And, fathers, provoke not your children to wrath: but bring them up in the nurture and admonition of the Lord" (Ephesians 6:4). Incorrectly applied discipline is stressful on parents and children alike.

Scripture offers numerous parables about disciplining disobedient children. Corporal punishment, administered properly, remains one means of correction. At the same time, some children respond very poorly to spanking, especially if the parent is angry when handing out the punishment. Other methods are often effective, such as invoking a "time out" in which the child is isolated for a period to reflect on wrongdoing.

Consistency is vital for effective discipline. Application of correction should not vary widely from child to child or occurrence to occurrence. At the same time, parents should recognize the unique differences between children.

Sometimes the best correction is verbal; at other times, children need corporal punishment. In all situations, parents should talk with their children about what was done, why it was wrong, how the action has hurt others, and what needs to be done to correct the situation. In some cases, discipline involves cleaning up a mess, apologizing for angry words, or helping someone else.

Another key to discipline is unity between parents. Parents should support one another when they have to correct a child. When possible, Mom and Dad will want to talk about how to handle disobedience. Where conferences are not possible, the absent parent should trust the best judgment of the disciplining parent and not allow the child to play one against the other. If parents differ greatly on how to discipline, they may experience stress in their own relationship. In no case should they play out their disagreements in front of the child.

A final consideration involves correcting attitudes versus behavior. Certainly, improper conduct needs discipline. Of greater importance, however, are attitudes behind the actions. If parents merely respond in kind to disrespectful words, facial expressions, body language, or other evidence of rebellious attitudes, they merely lower themselves to the child's level. After all, someone has to be the grownup!

Ultimately, parents want to move from mere discipline to discipling. They will have much greater long-term success by building into their children the desire to please God and follow His Word than just correcting misdeeds. God has called us to make disciples of all people. Disciple making begins with our own households. By setting the example, by teaching principles of life from God's Word, by pointing out benefits of good decisions and harmful effects of poor decisions, and other such tools of discipleship, we can build into our children the desire to follow the Lord and honor Him.

The Pain of Prodigals

Everyone who knew Bob and Sandy thought they were the ideal couple. They loved the Lord and their children. Coming to Christ as young adults, they had experienced difficulties prior to salvation but seemed to have moved forward in their Christian lives. That's why their children's behavior seemed so strange. Although raised in church with godly, loving parents, the children began to rebel as they hit high school. Over the years that followed, they experienced divorces, trouble holding jobs, and other problems. Throughout their prodigal years, their parents continued to love them, pray for them, and minister to them. Although their hearts ached for their kids, Bob and Sandy kept trusting God to bring them back to Him and to them.

Faithfully serving God does not mean children and teenagers will not follow the ways of the prodigal son. Just like the son who left home, demanding his father's inheritance while rejecting his father's values, some young people rebel against their parents and their God (Luke 15:11–32). Some prodigals have never been converted and follow the natural tendencies of lost adolescents. Others who have not been discipled may fall prey to bad influences from peers. Still others succumb to the temptations of the world, the flesh, or the devil, having chosen carnal lifestyles.

Pain produces pain. Many prodigals do not follow destructive patterns because they enjoy sin but act out of anger, fear, or pain. People who have been hurt tend to hurt others. Teens who become bitter often strike out at parents (or even at God). Pain inflicted by prodigals affects everyone around them. They also suffer from their own actions.

Parents experience pain from their prodigal's attitudes and actions. In his important work, *Parents in Pain: Overcoming the Hurt and Frustration of Problem Children*, John White observed that many parents struggle in their marriages when their children rebel. He notes that children can make a marriage stronger or tear it apart. Couples may struggle with each other, particularly when the mother and father disagree on the nature of the problem or the way toward solution. Their individual pain over their child's difficulties can be misdirected toward one another.[1]

Siblings also can be affected by prodigals' problems. Some children may feel confused over the tension in the family. Younger children who look up to their older brothers or sisters may be tempted to follow in their footsteps. Because the prodigal child becomes the focus of parental attention, other siblings may feel they are not as important. Like the elder son in the Prodigal Parable, they may become jealous when parents do more for the wayward siblings. They wonder, *We've been good. So, why do Mom and Dad seem to love Billy* (or Suzy or Tom or Jane) *more?*

Ruth Bell Graham (Mrs. Billy Graham) has shared her experiences with the pain of prodigals. From the struggles of her own children to her observations of other parents whose children wander, she wrote: "For some reason, they (prodigals) are usually thought of as teenage boys. But prodigals are not limited in gender. . . . They do have one thing in common: They have left home . . . and they are missed."[2]

Wait prayerfully. One way to respond to prodigals is merely to wait faithfully, watchfully, and prayerfully for their return. In her book, Mrs. Graham shared something of the heartache she and Dr. Graham endured waiting for their prodigals to come home. Yet the result was worth the wait. Like the prodigal in the parable, wayward children may eventually come to their senses and make their way home. In most cases, parents' investments of love and nurture will not prove fruitless (Proverbs 22:6).

The family's role in waiting is to pray and to trust God to work in their children's lives. God loves both parents and their children and will not abandon a lamb just because he or she has gone astray. Too, God's ear is not deafened to the cries of a heartsick mother or father who cries out to Him for their children. Richard Burr's book, *Praying Your Prodigal Home*, urges praying families to maintain faith in a loving heavenly Father Who is just as concerned about the prodigal as they. Effective prayers are rooted in faith, which in turn is founded on the Word of God, not mere wishes or emotions.[3] Burr also reminds praying parents to make sure their own hearts are right before the Lord.[4] One of the key aspects is forgiveness. If prodigals perceive only judgment and punishment await them, they may stay away.

James writes that prayer which avails much is fervent and comes from a righteous soul (James 5:16). Only when we bring our own sins under the blood and forgiveness of Christ can we pray effectively.

Wait expectantly. Another aspect of waiting is expecting. The father of the prodigal must have been in the habit of looking down the road where his son walked away. Perhaps, he gazed down that lane each day, wondering if that would be the day his son would come home. Do you suppose he became tired or discouraged when his son did not return after many days? Perhaps, but the father did not give up and neither should you. Have faith and wait patiently on the Lord.

Sometimes parents want to rescue their children. The prodigals' sins put them in difficult and even dangerous situations. The son of the parable lost all his money and became so hungry he took on a job no Jewish boy could imagine—tending pigs. He was so down and out he would have eaten the stuff the pigs were eating. What might have happened if the father had kept sending him money? Would this young man ever have come to his senses if his sin was rewarded by Dad getting him out of trouble every time God brought discipline into his life?

God loves us enough to bring us to a point of brokenness. Only through repentance—a change of mind that results in a change of life—can sinners (us included) find their way back to God. Sometimes it takes brokenness for us to experience repentance. At the same time, parents may need to intervene if their prodigals experience genuine danger. They may have fallen so far they cannot help themselves. They may want desperately for the parents to come and get them.

Years ago, I received a call from a minister who needed help finding an eighteen-year-old daughter of one of his parishioners. The girl had run away from home and made her way to a large city where I was serving. Thousands of young people lived on the streets because they felt anything was better than the restrictions of their home life. Being an adult, only she could choose to go back home. I found her and tried to show her how much her parents missed her and wanted her to return. Her curt reply was, "If they loved me so much, why didn't they come get me instead of sending you?" Calling the parents, I encouraged them to do what was necessary to reach out to their daughter with love and redemption.

Persevere in spiritual warfare. Although often rejected, families of prodigals must persevere in prayer if they wish to prevail in the spiritual battle for their children. Quin Sherrer and Ruthanne Garlock chronicle the lives of numerous prodigals who ultimately returned to Christ and to their families. A consistent aspect of their strategy is consistent, fervent prayer. They advise, ". . . We must carry the prayer burden until we see results." Their approach to *Praying Prodigals Home* recognizes the ultimate enemy is Satan who has stolen precious lives. Families must engage in powerful spiritual warfare through prayer to "take back what the Enemy has stolen."[5]

Provide a welcoming home. Many prodigals hesitate to return home for fear they will be rejected. The father in the parable greeted his son with a hug, a robe (covering his shame), and a ring (a sign of assurance he was not a servant, but a son). When prodigals return, the entire family needs to open their arms to the returning wanderer. Siblings who feel wounded by the prodigal's actions may resent the welcome that parents give the sinner. Jesus' story reminds the family that they are no longer prodigals; they are brothers and sisters, sons and daughters.

Some prodigals may never respond, no matter how much love and prayer are offered. A few prodigals may not find their way back. Many, however, will wake up one day and realize how much they left behind. They have a family that loves them and waits for them. They have a heavenly Father Who is willing to forgive and restore them. One day, waiting fathers and mothers will look down the lane and see the glad sight of a prodigal making his, or her, way home.

Chapter Seven
WHO WILL TAKE CARE OF ME?

Help for Caregivers

The funeral was bittersweet. Sadie wept as the minister spoke of her mother's life. Sadie's mom, Tanya, had been a wonderful woman. She took care of her family, worked hard to maintain a successful business, and ministered to countless of people in many ways. As Tanya reached advanced years, her physical health began to give way and Sadie, who was by now single herself, moved in to take care of her mom. For several years, she balanced her work with responsibilities related to her mother's care.

After Tanya suffered a series of strokes, additional difficulties multiplied the emotional and physical load Sadie bore. Her mom could no longer communicate, and caregiving became even more stressful. Sadie grieved over her mother's struggle to speak. Another challenge was Tanya's inability to get to the bathroom or even use a portable toilet. Sadie silently dealt with the practical issues of sanitation and tried to help her mother maintain a level of dignity in the process.

When Tanya died, Sadie grieved as anyone else would over the loss of a mother. At the same time, her years of constant caregiving were over. She had not been able to enjoy a personal life for a long time. Unable to leave her mom alone, she remained at the house unless a relative could come and relieve her for a short while so she could go to the grocery store or handle other errands.

Now she found herself free. A sense of relief brought with it a perplexing reaction of guilt. She was amazed at herself for feeling happy that she no longer had the constant burden of caregiving. Yet, she truly missed her mom and grieved over her death. These conflicting emotions are not uncommon for caregivers. Sadie would need some time and perhaps some godly counsel to make the difficult transition to her new life.

People who have not been the primary caregivers for someone who needs constant attention cannot fully appreciate how one's life becomes centered on the person needing care. Other needs are set aside. Vacations and days off may be difficult or impossible. Your mental and emotional focus, as well as your physical presence and effort, become centered on the person in need.

The urgency of the immediate makes us excuse setting aside the demands of other aspects of life, even the needs of other people in our lives. We feel guilty if we take time for ourselves. Should we begin to harbor resentment of our situation, feeling trapped by our circumstance, we experience conflicted emotions. We love the person we are caring for, but we hate the inability to get on with regular life, and then we feel guilty for thinking that way.

The Settings of Caregiving

Caregiving has many different portraits, but all have similar demands that produce varying levels of stress. Consider just a few:

Child-Rearing

Raising children is a normal type of caregiving that every family experiences. Parents go through the developmental stages of their kids' growth—from dealing with diapers to potty training. They tend to skinned knees when the infants try to walk and again when the six-year-old tries to ride a bicycle for the first time. They watch children struggle with schoolwork and schoolmates. They try to help mend children's broken toys and teenagers' broken hearts. Even after the kids have grown up and have families of their own, parents do not end their worry. They just extend their concern to another generation and start the cycle over again.

Physical Problems

Short-term illness. All families deal with illness. Most of the time, parents find themselves stressed over the typical sicknesses children experience. What mother, or father for that matter, has not spent long hours bathing a fevered brow with a wet cloth to reduce fever? What parent has found a secret to getting medicine in the middle of the night when all the pharmacies are closed?

Occasionally, parents get sick and have the double stress of managing their own illness as well as making sure someone gets the kids dressed, fed, and off to school on time. In the case of single parents, the load becomes especially hard. Extended family and friends can help. If someone does not have relatives living close enough to provide assistance, the church should be sensitive and offer to meet some of these needs.

Chronic illness. People who have not suffered chronic illness cannot fully understand the debilitating stress that often accompanies long-term suffering. When a problem has a possible resolution, hope gives the patient and his or her family courage to endure. Without the knowledge that a light indeed exists and the tunnel does eventually end, people can be tempted to fall into despair. Some chronic illnesses are not life threatening, but they create constant pain. Many medications often have side effects or grow less effective over time. Sufferers may sense they cannot escape the ever-present discomfort.

Permanent handicaps. I never thought of my great aunt as being handicapped. Following an auto accident when she was sixteen, she was unable to use her legs. Her parents had to use a hoist to get her in and out of bed. She needed help in many ways. I always knew her with the wheelchair, but her positive attitude and loving spirit never suggested she struggled with her condition. When her parents died, she moved into an assisted-living facility, where she also worked for many years. She taught me that even with permanent handicaps, a person can have a productive and healthy life.

Through the years, I've been blessed to know a number of people whose faith gave them strength to overcome their disabilities. Two young girls who suffered multiple congenital problems were vibrant examples of courage and grace. A young man with Down's syndrome always had a smile on his face, regardless of his health. Other special people have inspired me and everyone who knew them.

At the same time, both the handicapped persons and their families experience daily stresses. Needing help with a range of daily needs, they depend on others for basic necessities. Families may struggle with the physical and financial issues required to provide ongoing care. Relatives and friends can help to a degree. The church also should offer assistance, whether through spiritual counsel, financial help, or other ways. Still, the ongoing demands of such situations produce various levels of stress on the individuals and their families.

Mental Challenges

Special needs children. Bill and Maude loved their son. Freddie was special in many ways. He was born when Bill and Maude had already reached middle age. Unable to have children for many years, they had given up hope that they could ever enjoy the blessings of little feet running around the house. Then Freddie came along. Their elation changed to sorrow after they discovered Freddie would always be mentally challenged. He was happy and loving, but he would never be able to have a normal life. He would always need someone to take care of him. Bill and Maude were glad to meet his needs but worried what would happen to him when they died.

At first they blamed themselves for Freddie's condition. Although rarely at fault, caregivers often feel guilt for their loved ones' difficulties. Bill and Maude questioned whether they should have continued trying to have children. They worried that something they did might have resulted in Freddie's problem. Finally, they accepted that God had given Freddie to them to be as much a blessing for them as they could be to him. They embraced their role with joy. While the demands of caring for Freddie produced elements of stress along the way, they learned to manage their own challenges while caring for his.

Aging adults. On the other end of the spectrum, Carrie and her husband, Tom, found themselves in long discussions about what they would do with Charlie, her dad. Carrie's mother had died the previous year, and her father was showing increasing evidence of advanced Alzheimer 's disease. They no longer joked about his chronic forgetfulness. At times, Charlie did not recognize family members. He became confused about where he was, even questioning whether his house was really the place where he lived. On a couple of occasions, he had wandered away from home, setting off a frantic search by family and friends until he was found. Unable to prepare meals or care for himself, Charlie could not remain at home alone.

Carrie and Tom discussed options. They did not have the financial resources for an assisted-care facility and did not want to commit Charlie to a nursing home. Yet, they both had jobs they depended on to meet their own needs. On top of it all, their daughter had just given birth to twins and needed Carrie's help. They both loved Carrie's father, but struggled to find a solution for his care.

On the other side of town, Suzy was also wrestling with the stress of caregiving. Her husband, Leroy, had developed Parkinson's disease. In addition, he had started showing signs of dementia. They had the financial means to get medical help, but Suzy wanted to take care of Leroy at home. On most days, they enjoyed a quiet life in a semi-retired setting. However, other days were heartbreaking as Leroy grappled with his deteriorating physical abilities and as Suzy struggled with his increasing mental complications.

The Stress of Caregiving

An entire book could be written about the challenges of caregiving. Each situation carries unique sets of stressors that weigh on people who care for other people. If you ask them, most caregivers will discount their own discomfort because they view their personal sacrifice as minimal when compared with the problems experienced by the ones for whom they care. Still, if caregivers ignore their own needs, they can find themselves unable to provide the kind of help their loved ones require. Caregivers and those who care for the caregiver must take steps to manage their stress.

Here are just a few areas in which caregivers must attend to their own needs:

Riding the Emotional Roller Coaster

The very fact that we love the ones to whom we minister adds a depth of emotional stress. Caring people hurt when they see their loved ones suffer. A pain observed is a pain experienced. When we skinned our knees as children, Mother could make the hurt go away with a kiss. It's too bad the hurts of life cannot be as easily healed. We see people wounded by illness, accident, or age and we want to help them be better somehow, but often we can only bind up their bodies and succor their suffering. That hurts. We are in pain because we cannot totally relieve their discomfort.

Because the caregiver's emotions are closely tied to the well-being of their patient, an inevitable rise and fall of feelings follow the cycles of improvement and decline. Hope leaps in a caregiver's heart when the patient shows signs of regaining strength but crashes as the mountaintops of recovery yield to valleys of deterioration.

Some caregivers will battle conflicting emotions. They may approach exhaustion as stress builds and ongoing demands of the patient's condition draw deep on the reserves of everyone's strength. Anger over the patient's condition can be directed at the illness itself, or at perceived inability by physicians to achieve healing, or even at God for the lack of answered prayer. Left unattended, the caregiver can grow bitter even toward the patient, an unacceptable emotion that results in the caregiver struggling with guilt. Depression can set in if solutions are not implemented.

One of my friends spent many years caring for his wife, a victim of Alzheimer's disease. Finding himself wrestling physically, emotionally, and spiritually, he sought the advice of a godly physician. The doctor's observation was that my friend was experiencing many of the same symptoms that characterize victims of Post-Traumatic Stress Disorder. Indeed, a chronic caregiver can suffer trauma from long years of watching a loved one suffer, producing significant personal pain along the way.

Certainly, not all caregiving casts so dire a shadow. Quite often the ministration of loving care receives the blessing of recovery and health. Caregivers need the anticipation that things can indeed get better and an end is in sight. Still, even in the best situations, during the crisis itself the caregiver can experience a wide range of emotional stress.

Finding the Finances

Most people are not fully prepared for the financial demands extended caregiving presents. A lifetime of savings can evaporate with just a few large medical procedures lying outside the coverage of insurance. Long-term care policies can help but do not cover all the extra costs involved, particularly if a family chooses to care for the patient in their home. Special dietary needs, medication, expensive equipment, and trips to the hospital and doctors' offices are just a few of the matters that drain a family's resources. Additionally, the caregiver may have to take off from work, resulting in a loss of needed income just when expenses spiral upward.

Balancing Demands

Time is a nonrenewable resource. Most people already have their schedule, and their budget, allotted to existing commitments. They are not prepared for the extra demands on time, attention, and resources that emergency care requires. Whether a short-term illness that takes a child out of school or a long-term condition that demands extended attention, we seldom have the luxury of setting aside other obligations easily.

The other children have to get to school and then to band practice and then to Suzy's birthday party, and a hundred other activities. Meals have to be prepared. The car breaks down. The boss wants that report completed by the end of the week. The work has been promised and cannot be postponed. Caregivers may be blessed with generous supervisors who grant emergency leave for family emergencies, but most companies have limits as to how many days they can give without the worker's job being in jeopardy.

Taking care of hurting loved ones, whether over a short or long term, present a virtual juggling act for conscientious families. Hopefully, everyone will pitch in and help, but the primary caregiver always senses the ultimate responsibility, and with it the stress, of making it all work out.

Help for Hurting Hearts

Most caregivers are altruistic by nature and rarely consider their own needs. The first is an honorable trait; the second is a horrible mistake. Being others-focused is a character quality we all should desire. However, if caregivers do not take care of themselves or allow others to minister to help them, they can find themselves unable to care for their patients. Constantly giving and never receiving, they soon become exhausted physically, mentally, emotionally, and spiritually.

Here are several actions caregivers can undertake to insure they have the personal resources to function effectively:

Pray

Most Christian caregivers are people of faith. They believe in God, and they believe He hears their prayers. So they pray. Certainly they should pray for the loved one who rests in their care. Nothing is wrong with asking the Great Physician to heal, the Holy Comforter to comfort, or the heavenly Father to help.

Yet, caregivers also need to pray for themselves. It is not selfish to pray for strength, grace, wisdom, rest, resources, or any of the countless other needs a caregiver experiences. Jesus encourages us to ask the Father in the Son's Name: "Hitherto have ye asked nothing in my name: ask, and ye shall receive, that your joy may be full" (John 16:24).

Still, effective prayer involves bringing our needs before the Lord and taking time each day with the Lord in personal communion. Much of the caregiver's stress comes from having one's life focused on the patient's needs, which can become overwhelming. By spending time in communion with Christ, we are able to retreat into His presence, receive His love, and refresh ourselves with His Spirit. Learn to abide in Him in those moments of private prayer as well as in the busyness of caregiving. Look up and find Him present with you at the bedside. You will find no place to go, no task to do, no difficulty to overcome that He is not there with you. Remember, ". . . He hath said, I will never leave thee, nor forsake thee. So that we may boldly say, The Lord *is* my helper, . . ." (Hebrews 13:5–6).

Ask for Help and Accept What's Offered

One of life's ironies involves our reluctance to ask for or accept help when we need it the most. Friends, family members, and church members may have sincerely good intentions when they say, "Let me know if I can help in any way." However, the general nature of their offer leaves us not wanting to impose on them. Consequently, we continue to struggle, and they miss out on a blessing because we deny them the opportunity to come alongside us in caregiving.

In Galatians 6:5, Paul acknowledged the importance of each person bearing his own burden. The word for *burden* in this case is the ordinary responsibilities of life. However, in verse 2, Paul encouraged believers to bear one another's burdens. He employed a different word for *burden*. This reference involves an overwhelming burden, one so heavy it would crush the average person. Caregivers should allow other people to help them bear the overpowering loads of life.

Have Some Standby's

Closely related to the above admonition, keep some people on standby. You never know when you need to run to the grocery store or pharmacy. An emergency may come up with your other children that requires you to leave the patient and go to the school. Sometimes, you just need to get out of the house or away from the hospital for a while. If your patient cannot be left alone, having some relatives, friends, or church colleagues available can give you the peace of mind that your loved one is in good care.

Make Use of External Resources

Caregivers have numerous resources outside themselves and their family to help care for their patients. If you bring the person home from the hospital but need additional medical help, talk to the hospital social worker to see about using a home health care agency. My ninety-four-year-old mother-in-law was greatly helped by such an organization. They provided an electronic home monitoring unit, physical therapy, someone to help provide a bath, and a nurse for two months after she came home

129

from the hospital. In some situations, insurance or Medicare programs may provide hospital-type beds, oxygen, or other equipment to help you provide care at home.

Sleep When You Can

Caring for someone in your home or at the hospital often means nights filled with constant interruptions. A patient's needs do not shut off like a light switch just because it is bedtime. Sleep deprivation can be deadly. If you cannot find someone to sit with the patient during the night, you may have to find ways to sleep when you can during the day. Yet, sleep you must. After only a few days without proper rest, you will find yourself experiencing serious physical problems of your own. Stress becomes much more intense in its effects without proper sleep. If your patient is sleeping, take a nap—even if it's the middle of the day.

Eat Well

Meals can be another challenge for caregivers. If the stress lingers and grows in severity, you may find yourself unable to eat. You may simply feel too tired to prepare a balanced, nutritious meal. Junk food, fast food, and comfort food help you get past the immediate cravings but are counterproductive in giving you the physical strength needed for your ongoing task. Make personal health a priority not only for your own sake and that of the rest of your family but for your patient.

Take a Walk

Find some way to exercise on a regular basis. You may not find time to go down to the local gym, but you can take a walk. Even a short walk around the yard or down the street will get you out of the house. Breathe in some fresh air. Bask in the sunshine. Look around and see beauty where you can find it. Having exercise equipment is helpful during rainy or cold days, but a brisk walk outside can work wonders for handling stress.

Talk to Someone

Caregiving can be a lonely endeavor, if you let it. Your heart fills with worries, doubts, fears, and a hundred other emotions. While some people talk freely about their problems, others internalize their feelings. Holding negative thoughts inside rarely produces a good result. Talk with someone about your feelings, your experience, and your needs. Find a confidante with whom you can share the secrets of your heart. If not in person, use the phone. Even before you feel the pressure overloading, use the release valve of conversation to relieve the stress. The person you talk with may not offer any answers, but simply having someone to share your heart is healthy.

Be careful about using social media to share personal matters. Too many people are stalking the cyberspace looking for vulnerable targets. Having said that, sharing prayer needs with friends can produce a wave of intercession just when you need it.

Take Time

Along the way, take time each day—for yourself, for God, and for others in your life. Everyone needs to get alone and be quiet for a while. The stress of noise (with crying babies), or smells (with incontinent patients), or pain wears on the strongest of caregivers. Getting by yourself, even for a few minutes, can help you relax and settle your emotions. If you are concerned about hearing the patient call if a need arises, buy a set of baby monitors. Even if the patient is elderly, monitors are an inexpensive way to give you the ability to hear or see what is going on while doing something else.

Home monitoring systems help caregivers be away from the house without constant worry about the patient being unable to summon help. Several companies rent devices that provide a button an elderly person can press for emergency assistance. If you have to be away from the house, having such a system in place gives you confidence that even if someone is unable to call you on the phone, all he or she has to do is press a button and help will come. These systems usually include smoke detecting. Responders notify the person responsible for the patient's care, as well as EMT, fire, police, or any other needed party.

Finally, be sure to take time for the other people in your life. Try not to allow your children, spouse, or others become jealous of your love, time, and attention. Sharing your time with others ministers to them and helps you. You benefit by healthy relationships with family and friends.

At its best, caregiving involves many different sources of stress. Gratefully, God gives us numerous resources to manage the pressure of personal ministry. Through His help, with His strength, and by His grace, caregivers can bless the lives of hurting people and thrive personally in the process.

Chapter Eight
WHAT'S THE PROBLEM?

Reducing Stress through Conflict Resolution

"As much as it lies within you, live peaceably with all men" (Romans 12:18).

Conflict produces more stress than nearly anything else in our lives. No one likes conflict. Most people prefer positive, mutually encouraging relationships, but conflict interrupts our lives in spite of our best intentions. Conflict may center on task issues—what to do and how to do it. Conflict also arises from interactions between various personality types.

Conflict commonly occurs between people in close proximity. That's one reason we see so much conflict within the average home. Even Christian families experience sibling rivalry, arguments over toys, conflict over personal space, and much more. Husbands and wives disagree over money, decisions, sex, and many other issues. Teenagers and parents find they have trouble understanding one another, often arguing about rules and discipline. This constant friction in the family requires deliberate approaches to achieve resolution and peace in the home.

The best way to resolve conflict is to avoid it. By demonstrating the fruit of the Spirit in our relationships, we are more likely to provoke positive responses. Generally, people will react well if we are loving instead of hateful, joyful rather than sour, peaceful rather than combative, patient rather than short tempered, gentle rather than rough, good rather than evil, faithful rather than undependable, meek rather than arrogant, and temperate rather than self-indulgent (Galatians 5:16–23).

If we incorporate spiritual wisdom into our relationships, we can avoid much sorrow. Avoiding attitudes and actions that hurt others stops the fire before it starts. At the same time, we should cultivate those behaviors that build up the relationship. As we follow the model our Savior gave in His life and in His teaching, we can live in love rather than conflict.

Reconciliation Is Vital to Christian Relationships

"And all things are of God, who has reconciled us to himself by Jesus Christ, and has given to us the ministry of reconciliation; To wit, that God was in Christ, reconciling the world unto Himself, not imputing their trespasses unto them; and has committed unto us the word of reconciliation. Now then we are ambassadors for Christ, as though God did beseech you by us: we pray you in Christ's stead, be reconciled to God" (2 Corinthians 5:18–20).

We have a responsibility and opportunity to initiate reconciliation. Believers are the recipients of His gracious work of reconciliation, bringing us into a right relationship with Him through Jesus. As such, each believer has received a ministry of reconciliation, beginning with our own families. The foundation of the ministry of reconciliation is the word of reconciliation: ". . . that God was in Christ, reconciling the world unto Himself . . ." (2 Corinthians 5:19). The basis by which we can help resolve interpersonal conflict is God's atoning work in Christ.

Reconciliation begins with Christ, then one another. Only Jesus can bring true peace within one's heart and between His people (John 14:27). Mediators who work with believers should begin by talking about their relationship with Christ. Jesus in one person cannot be in conflict with Jesus within another person. Where conflict exists, one or more of the parties have stepped away from a committed and submitted relationship to the Lord. Bringing each person closer to Christ, by nature, results in their coming closer to one another. Scripture provides the strongest common ground for people to experience reconciliation.

"... as though God did beseech you by us: we pray you in Christ's stead, be reconciled to God" (2 Corinthians 5:20).

Being peacemakers identifies us as children of God. Jesus is the Prince of Peace (Isaiah 9:6). We show ourselves to be His children and experience His blessing when we engage in making peace (Matthew 5:9). Disliking conflict, we may shy away from intervening into other people's conflicts, but such is the ministry He has given us. Much more, when we are part of the conflict, we cannot escape our responsibility to join Jesus in the work of peacemaking.

When conflict happens despite the best efforts, what can we do to resolve the disagreement and, in doing so, reduce the stress? Proverbs 20:3 reminds us "It is an honor for a man to cease from strife: but every fool will be meddling." So, what should you do if you find yourself in conflict?

Resolving Interpersonal Conflict

Following are some steps you can take to reduce stress by resolving conflict. However, not every situation follows a nice, step-by-step process. Each relationship is different. How you handle conflict within the family and how you resolve issues with people outside the family will vary. These ideas are biblical principles that can guide you in making peace with others. You probably will not use all of these steps in each occasion, nor will you employ them in the same order as listed. Still, I think you will find help in building healthy relationships.

Communicate

This first point is not numbered because it is necessary for all of the steps that follow. People in conflict tend to disagree, argue, fuss, and fight until they get to a certain level of anger, at which point they cut off communication altogether. Arguments can be worked out if people are still talking. Once someone stops communicating, you will find it difficult to resolve a conflict.

Communicate honestly. Too many people conceal their true feelings or desires. When engaged in disagreements, they may simply say, "It's okay" when matters are really not okay at all. They may have developed habits of hiding their emotions during childhood years. They could be afraid to share their thoughts. However, if people do not honestly communicate, they rarely resolve problems. At the same time, we should never justify saying something in a mean way by using the excuse, "I'm just being honest."

Communicate politely. Don't be afraid to share your point of view as long as you do so kindly. People in conflict often allow their emotions to control their tongues. Scripture warns about the problems of unguarded speech. Jesus warned against angry words, as did James (Matthew 5:22; James 1:9). We can learn to share our feelings and thoughts without doing so in an offensive way. If we value the other person and want to heal the relationship, we will speak politely. Remember what we've already noted: "A soft answer turns aside wrath" (Proverbs 15:1).

Have a discussion, not a monologue. Speaking to be heard or to force someone to accept our point of view rarely resolves differences. A two-way discussion requires both parties to respect each other, even if they are in conflict. They must want to understand each other.

Listen before you speak. Too often, while the other person is talking, we are not listening; we are forming what we plan to say in response. Scripture advises: "He that answers a matter before he hears it, it is folly and shame unto him" (Proverbs 18:13).

Use active listening to make sure you understand what the other person is saying. Ask open-ended questions to encourage the person to share his or her point of view. Clarify statements by repeating the person's statements and then asking, "Am I understanding you correctly?" Listen for what's not being said as much as for what is said. Watch for clues from the person's body language, tone of voice, and other nonverbal variables to gauge emotions or discover unspoken issues.

Keeping in mind the absolute necessity for good communication, consider the following tips for conflict resolution:

1. Honestly examine yourself.

Jesus said we should examine our hearts before we attempt to correct someone else: "And why do you behold the speck that is in thy brother's eye, but perceive not the beam that is in your own eye? Either how can you say to your brother, 'Brother, let me pull out the speck that is in your eye,' when you do not see the beam that is in your own eye? You hypocrite, cast out first the beam out of your own eye, and then you will see clearly to pull out the speck that is in your brother's eye" (Luke 6:41–42).

Honestly ask yourself if you are at fault in some way. Have you said or done something to provoke the dispute? Have you exhibited an attitude that offended the other person? Do you really love this person and want the best for him/her?

One mother disciplined her child for his explosion of anger against his brother. Afterward, she realized she was guilty of the same offense by exercising discipline out of anger rather than correction. Humbling herself, she confessed the sin to God and her child. She went further and imposed the same punishment on herself that she had used on her child. Her attitude and action had a strong effect on her son. He had a greater respect for her and better understanding of how he should behave in the future.

2. Lovingly understand the other person.

Do you understand what problems they may be dealing with at work, in the home, or personally? It may be that the conflict you are experiencing is actually fallout from conflict or difficulties in other places, producing stress that carries over into other relationships.

Could you be experiencing a cross-personality conflict? As mentioned earlier, various personality types have difficulty understanding and relating to certain other types. Have you considered that each person has approached an issue from particularly personality perspectives?

In a retreat, I taught a group of couples how the DISC personality profiles work and how the different personalities can complement one another instead of conflicting. After the presentation, one husband and wife approached me and shared how they had been on the verge of divorce for many years. After the presentation, they finally understood how they had allowed their personalities to conflict instead of helping one another. With a greater appreciation of how God had made each of them, they committed to build a stronger relationship that would honor Him.

Have you wondered what people want from you and whether such expectations are legitimate? Does someone think that you have not lived up to a perceived agreement? Or vice versa? Have you prayed about the person's relationship with the Lord? People who are not right with God will not be right with people. On the other hand, "When a man's ways please the LORD, he makes even his enemies to be at peace with him" (Proverbs 16:7).

3. Do not be quick to judge.

Take time to listen and understand. Too often, we tend to jump to judgment. Instead of wisely listening to all sides to a dispute, we offer quick fixes that usually do more harm than good. As we've mentioned before, "He who answers a matter before he hears it, it is folly and shame to him" (Proverbs 18:13). Peacemakers invest sufficient time to understand what is actually going on before trying to solve the problem.

Recognize your liability. Don't be quick to judge because we all will be judged. "But why do you judge your brother? Or why do you set at naught your brother? For we shall all stand before the judgment seat of Christ" (Romans 14:10).

Be fair. If we expect others to do what is right, we must be fair in handling all conflicts. We, too, have a Judge Who will utilize whatever standard of judgment we have employed with others. "Judge not, that you be not judged. For with what judgment you judge, you shall be judged: and with what standard you measure, it shall be measured to you again" (Matthew 7:1–2).

Employ wise discernment. Avoiding being judgmental does not mean we cannot be discerning. Maintaining order requires us to use godly wisdom in determining the truth when fellow believers have disagreements. "Dare any of you, having a matter against another, go to law before the unjust, and not before the saints? Do ye not know that the saints shall judge the world? and if the world shall be judged by you, are ye unworthy to judge the smallest matters? Know ye not that we shall judge angels? how much more things that pertain to this life?" (1 Corinthians 6:1–3).

Avoid a spirit of condemnation. Attitudes can make or break conflict resolution. If we approach others with a spirit of condemnation, we not only will fail to achieve reconciliation, but we also put ourselves in danger of judgment and condemnation. "Judge not, and you shall not be judged: condemn not, and you shall not be condemned: forgive, and you shall be forgiven" (Luke 6:37).

4. Wisely discern the real issues behind the conflict.

Identify evidence of sin at the root of conflict. "From whence come wars and fighting among you? Come they not hence, even of your lusts that war in your members?" (James 4:1). Too often, people in conflict focus on assigning blame instead of resolving the problem. Everyone involved in a problem should humbly search their hearts to discern whether sinful desires are at the root of the fight. If the other person is at fault, love him/her enough to deal with the issue in a humble manner (Galatians 6:1).

Is one of the parties to the conflict fearful of losing self-esteem? I spoke with one man who had become engaged in a terrible conflict with a colleague at his workplace. The issue seemed so trivial I asked why he had not merely yielded for the sake of the relationship. He answered that he felt he would lose his place of leadership if he let the other person win. He would rather risk ruining a relationship than appear not to be in control. Granted, some situations require courageous stands against evil. However, this situation came down to one matter—pride.

Some disagreements relate to generational perceptions and values. Various age groups approach decisions differently. The environmental influences of their generations often develop values that differ greatly from other age groups. For example, the builder generation (older people, many of whom experienced the Great Depression) are fearful of debt and tend to be very frugal. Younger adults grew up on credit and are only interested in whether they can make the payments. When a decision relates to financial questions, these two generations will approach solutions from very different perspectives.

Past experiences may shape a person's attitude. The person in conflict with you may see in you some aspect of another person who offended them in the past. In such cases, you have to help people open up about previous conflicts, show them you are not that person and this is not the same situation, and aid their coming to peace with their past so they might be at peace with their present.

Pain also influences people's reactions to situations and other people who may have nothing to do with the pain. Terry and Sam experienced constant conflict in meetings at their business. It seemed that no matter what one of them did or said, the other took the opposite position, often using strong emotion to insist on his point. Later, Terry discovered that his colleague was experiencing several painful situations. Their employer was downsizing the business, creating fear that people may lose their jobs. Sam's son had become very rebellious and started using drugs. Sam was also suffering from a health problem that potentially could become life threatening. His personal pain did not excuse his behavior, but understanding it enabled the two men to relate to one another differently.

Some conflicts relate to task issues, while other problems are personal. Understand whether the disagreement is over how to accomplish a particular task or if the conflict has taken on a personal nature. People-oriented conflict is much more difficult to resolve and requires different approaches.

5. **Try to limit the number of persons involved in the matter.**

Scripture advises anyone involved in conflict to approach the other person privately. "Moreover if your brother shall trespass against you, go and tell him his fault between you and him alone: if he shall hear you, you have gained your brother" (Matthew 18:15). The more people that are involved, the more difficult the resolution becomes. Pride rises. Sides are drawn. Advice starts flying from everyone at once, often without much wisdom, prayer, or seeking of scriptural guidance. Too, peer pressure and the herd mentality are very real, creating an intractable situation.

6. Remember what is at stake.

Who wins or loses is not as important as the honor and glory of God. When Christians fight, they dishonor the name of the One they claim as Lord. Jesus said, "By this shall all men know that you are my disciples, if you have love one for another" (John 13:35). This is especially true in the Christian home. In dealing with disagreements, all parties need to consider the effect that their dispute has on God's reputation.

Moreover, lost people often judge Christ on the basis of Christians' behavior. Does the community know you as people who love one another or as persons who cannot even be in right relationship with one another?

7. Are you a participant or a peacemaker?

Are you involved in the conflict or can you approach the problem as a third party whose only desire is to honor God? If you are a participant, you may need to seek a mediator who can help resolve the situation. Jesus taught that if one cannot resolve an issue privately, then ". . . take with you one or two more, that in the mouth of two or three witnesses every word may be established" (Matthew 18:16.) The witnesses are not there to take one side against the other. Rather, they are able to view both points of view impartially and mediate a resolution. In any case, they can testify to what is actually said and done between the conflicted parties.

Avoid being drawn into someone else's fight. Some people will share a problem with you, expecting you to set the other person straight. Their battle becomes yours and they often retire to the sidelines without responsibility for resolution or results, leaving you to suffer the scars that ensue. On the other hand, if you refuse to play their game, they may begin to perceive you as part of the problem and seek other people to take up their cause, often against you!

Sometimes you need to stand up for others. Especially when injustice is occurring or someone who is weaker is being bullied. The next chapter addresses this type of situation more fully. Be willing to defend people who are not able to fend for themselves.

8. Take the initiative to resolve the conflict, regardless of who is at fault.

People in conflict may be fearful of approaching others with whom they have conflict. Scripture reminds us that perfect love casts out fear. "There is no fear in love; but perfect love casts out fear: because fear hath torment. He that fears is not made perfect in love" (1 John 4:18). Prayerfully ask God to love the other person through you. When you come to the point of caring more for the other person than for your own pride or position, you are ready to initiate reconciliation and resolution.

Most people are willing to resolve conflict if the offender admits wrongdoing and asks forgiveness. Scripture does not give us the luxury of placing the responsibility for action on others. Regardless of who is at fault, we have the responsibility to initiate reconciliation.

If you have harmed someone, humbly admit the wrongdoing and ask for forgiveness. Confession may be difficult, particularly if you have been hurt by that person. Still, your responsibility is not what the other person may or may not do. You can only obey God's commandment for your actions. "Therefore if you bring your gift to the altar, and there remember that your brother has anything against you; Leave your gift before the altar, and go your way; first be reconciled to your brother, and then come and offer your gift" (Matthew 5:23–24).

Don't wait until the person at fault comes to you. I was sharing with a godly friend about a Christian leader who had wronged me. I said, "If he would just come and admit his wrong, we could be reconciled." My friend replied, "You have just identified the spiritual one in this problem." He pointed out Galatians 6:1. "Brothers, if a man be overtaken in a fault, you which are spiritual, restore such an one in the spirit of meekness; considering yourself, lest you also be tempted" (Galatians 6:1). I knew immediately that I had to call the other person and initiate reconciliation.

9. Pray together.

Put the matter in God's hand and seek to know the mind of Christ. It is hard to be angry with someone as you pray with them. In marriage counseling, I insist the husband and wife pray for one another as well as for the healing of their marriage. They pray aloud in the presence of each other. When they begin seeking God's best for each other, they are on their way to reconciliation.

10. Act.

Do not delay. Several practical reasons suggest you should take action as soon as the conflict becomes known:

- As time goes by, anger turns to bitterness, making resolution much more difficult.
- When conflict is caught early, most adversaries have not reached inflexible positions.
- If allowed to go unchecked, conflict draws other people like flies to trash, creating a much more complex situation.
- Conflict is like an infection; it rarely heals itself but only gets worse.

Scripture commands believers to act quickly to resolve disagreements:

- "Agree with your adversary quickly, while you are in the way with him; lest at any time the adversary delivers you to the judge, and the judge delivers you to the officer, and you are cast into prison" (Matthew 5:25). Whether the other person is at fault, or if we are wrong, the principle remains—work quickly to resolve the issue. Delayed reconciliation leads to escalation of the conflict, always causing more harm than the original problem.
- "Be ye angry, and sin not: let not the sun go down upon your wrath: Neither give place to the devil" (Ephesians 4:26–27). Delaying reconciliation prevents anger from being resolved. Allowed to go on unchecked, anger develops into bitterness. When we refuse to deal with our anger, we give the devil a platform within our hearts to attack our relationship with God and other people.

11. **Remain calm and speak gently.**

Remember the proverb: "A soft answer turns away wrath: but grievous words stir up anger" (Proverbs 15:1). Replacing anger with godly, Spirit-generated love allows you to respond to others with a humble heart. Instead of speaking with raised voice and strident spirit, you can speak in such a manner as to reduce the other person's anger. Once, a man angrily approached me about a matter. He stood up, raising his voice, and gesturing threateningly. Having grown up constantly fighting, my base nature was to stand and respond in kind. However, God gave grace, enabling me to remain seated, speaking in a low voice. The louder he got, the softer I spoke—not in fear but following the Spirit's leading. Soon, the man realized his anger was inappropriate. He sat down, lowered his voice, and allowed us to enter a genuine discussion of the issue. Reconciliation ended with both of us praying, thanking God for His grace.

12. **Lovingly rebuke wrongdoing.**

Going to other people does not mean you ignore their wrongdoing. "Take heed to yourselves: If thy brother trespass against thee, rebuke him; and if he repent, forgive him" (Luke 17:3). The sense of the passage does not suggest a harsh accusation but a firm admonishment. You may express strong disapproval, yet do so in a loving and gentle manner, remembering your own shortcomings (Galatians 6:1).

13. **Beware of holding grudges.**

Some personalities get mad easily but get over anger quickly. Others take time to boil over, yet retain grudges. Unfortunately, too many people blame their personality type for their unwillingness to deal with their lack of willingness to reconcile. Many people justify their bitterness by pointing out others' wrongdoing.

Believers have no excuse. We are more than the sum of our personalities because the Holy Spirit lives within us. We are responsible to submit to the scriptural admonition: "Grudge not one against another, brethren, lest you be condemned: behold, the judge stands before the door" (James 5:9).

14. Forgive and ask forgiveness.

Scripture admonishes us to rebuke offenders but equally commands us to forgive (Luke 17:3). Interestingly, many Christians talk about forgiveness but in practice are among the most reluctant to forgive. Throughout the New Testament, believers are admonished to forgive. Consider these passages:

- "Forbearing one another, and forgiving one another, if any man has a quarrel against any: even as Christ forgave you, so also do you" (Colossians 3:13). Christ has forgiven us such heinous sins that only His blood on the cross could make atonement. If He has forgiven us such great wrong, how can we refuse to forgive others? "And be kind one to another, tenderhearted, forgiving one another, even as God for Christ's sake hath forgiven you" (Ephesians 4:32).
- Sometimes we forgive, only to have the other person continue to harm us. At what point do we stop "turning the other cheek?" Jesus gives us the answer through His lesson to Peter: "Then came Peter to him, and said, Lord, how often shall my brother sin against me, and I forgive him? Till seven times? Jesus said unto him, I say not unto you, Until seven times: but, Until seventy times seven" (Matthew 18:21–22). Jesus told a parable of a man who owed much and was forgiven, only to be unforgiving toward a fellow servant who owed him a small amount. When other servants told the king, the unforgiving man was thrown into prison and his forgiven debt reissued. Jesus warned His followers: "So likewise shall my heavenly Father do also unto you, if you from your hearts forgive not everyone his brother their trespasses" (Matthew 18:35). The key phrase is "from the heart." We cannot give lip service to forgiveness; it must be totally genuine, without reservation.

- The only commentary Jesus offered about his Model Prayer was the phrase about forgiveness: "And forgive us our debts, as we forgive our debtors." Following the prayer, Jesus told His followers: "For if you forgive men their trespasses, your heavenly Father will also forgive you: But if you forgive not men their trespasses, neither will your Father forgive your trespasses" (Matthew 6:12–15). We may be uncomfortable with the idea that our forgiveness is tied to our willingness to forgive. Yet, Scripture offers this same admonishment not once, but several times.

- "And when you stand praying, forgive, if you have anything against any: that your Father also which is in heaven may forgive you your trespasses. But if you do not forgive, neither will your Father which is in heaven forgive your trespasses" (Mark 11:25–26).

- "Judge not, and you shall not be judged: condemn not, and you shall not be condemned: forgive, and you shall be forgiven" (Luke 6:37).

15. If you are wrong, admit it.

Confess your faults to the Lord and to the person you have offended. Scripture links healing to confession (James 5:16). Refusing to admit wrongdoing and resisting asking forgiveness increases internal stress. The other person becomes a source of stress because he or she reminds us of our guilt. Since we dislike the discomfort that stress produces, we tend to avoid those people who are parties to our conflict.

Denying our sin places us in the position of calling God a liar (1 John 1:10), but if we confess our sin, "He is faithful and just to forgive us our sin and cleanse us from all unrighteousness" (1 John 1:9). Just as confession and repentance are keys to reconciliation and forgiveness from God, we need to humble

> Ultimately, the most important outcome lies not in who wins or who gets his/her way but whether God is glorified.

ourselves to seek forgiveness from people we have offended (Matthew 5:23–24).

16. Emphasize God's honor.

In the end, the issue is not about us. When dealing with conflict, people tend to focus on themselves and the trouble. They may forget that how believers behave reflects on the name and reputation of God. Remind everyone involved that God's honor is at stake. Ultimately, the most important outcome lies not in who wins or who gets his/her way but whether God is glorified. Keeping the Lord's image in the forefront of the discussion motivates everyone to speak more kindly and to open themselves up to God's solution.

17. Find common ground.

During marriage counseling, I rarely begin by discussing the couple's problems. Talking about disagreements does not build a basis for healing wounded relationships. Instead, we talk about what attracted them to one another to begin with. As they recall good times and positive experiences, they recover common ground of the past on which to resolve current conflicts.

Common ground may involve agreement about issues. Before focusing on points of divergence, help each person to discover areas of agreement. At the famous Jerusalem Conference, the two sides came to the common agreement that God had brought salvation to the Gentiles just as He had to the Jews. The conditions of acceptance were agreeable to both parties. Peace was made and God was glorified (Acts 15).

Consulting with a church that was divided 60/40 on nearly all issues, I spent several weeks teaching about the importance of glorifying God in all things, including decisions about the church's future. In a series of meetings, we placed people around tables by random selection to force various parties to work together who had not been on speaking terms before. Tasking each table with deciding on five priorities for the church's future, but requiring unanimity before reporting to other groups, we left them to find common ground among themselves. After three weeks, each group shared their results. They discovered that they agreed on similar directions for the church after all. Having the first unanimous vote in years on those priorities led to ensuing joy and growth. Stress levels diminished as the people committed themselves to one another and to the glory of God.

18. Discuss issues and solutions honestly and respectfully.

Instead of imposing solutions on others, invite all parties to share their viewpoints. Sometimes, the basic problem relates to a misunderstanding of how each one perceives the situation. Encourage questions to address any confusion as to what speakers mean by various statements. Discourage attacks on personalities by keeping the attention focused on the issues.

During the discussion, ensure a fair hearing by everyone. Often people will go along with different ideas if they feel others are giving them a genuine opportunity to present their positions. As participants debate the problem and possible solutions, work to keep communication flowing. Once people stop talking honestly and freely, resolutions become nearly impossible.

19. Commit the situation and solutions to the Lord.

Sincerely seek God's direction, surrendering personal desires. The best resolution may be totally different than any that are proposed by participants. Search the Scriptures for principles that apply to the current problem. While specifics of the situation may be difficult to identify from biblical accounts, the Bible contains spiritual principles applied to every human dilemma.

Seek agreement in which people do not identify who wins or loses, but rather find a decision that glorifies Christ and, consequently, benefits His children. Such a result allows everyone to feel positively about the outcome and commit themselves to the ensuing direction.

What Do We Do if Conflict Is Not Resolved?

Jesus was the most Spirit-filled person ever to live, yet He constantly encountered opposition. In some situations, He resolved the conflict. In other places, He was rejected. In all cases, He loved the people involved, even when He rebuked them for their sin.

Sometimes conflict is unavoidable. You cannot control other people; you can only choose to behave in a peaceful, Christlike manner. Paul advised, "As much as it lies within you, live peaceably with all men" (Romans 12:18).

Give it Time

Some personalities get over personal pain quickly; others take much longer. The deeper and more emotional the hurt, the more time is required for healing. The old saying, "time heals all wounds" is not exactly correct, because time alone does not heal. Still, over a period of time, people become more open to healing and reconciliation. Give God time to work in your heart and in the lives of others involved in conflict. The Lord can heal and reconcile in an instant; however, people have to yield to His Spirit. Prayerfully and patiently wait for God's healing touch, opening your heart so, at least for your part, God can bring freedom.

Trust the Lord

When we swallow our pride and initiate actions to produce reconciliation, we expect action. We look for results immediately. If others do not respond quickly, we wonder if we have wasted our time; we are tempted to doubt God's willingness to work. Don't give up. Trust the Lord to fulfill His promises. He wants His children to live in harmony. Trust His willingness and His ability to work reconciliation in His timing.

Love in Spite of the Conflict

Do not fail to let God's grace continue to work. Keep bitterness from building a stronghold in your life. Instead, love the other person as Jesus has loved you. "A new commandment I give unto you, That ye love one another; as I have loved you, that ye also love one another" (John 13:34). Jesus did not wait to love us until we responded to His grace. "But God commends his love toward us, in that, while we were yet sinners, Christ died for us" (Romans 5:8).

What if the other person does not respond positively to your advances toward reconciliation? Jesus teaches us by precept and example to love people, even when they maintain hatred toward us: "But I say unto you, Love your enemies, bless them that curse you, do good to them that hate you, and pray for them which despitefully use you, and persecute you; That ye may be the children of your Father which is in heaven: for he makes his sun to rise on the evil and on the good, and sends rain on the just and on the unjust" (Matthew 5:44—45).

What about Church Discipline?

Church discipline rarely involves conflict resolution within a family. However, some situations may require the congregation to become involved for the good of the family as well as the church. If a couple considers divorce, especially because of sexual sin or other such problems, they would benefit in bringing the matter to the pastor for counseling. If the offender refuses to repent and be reconciled, wise and humble discipline by the congregation may help. Be careful at this point not to abuse the church's role by using others to get your way.

Matthew 18 teaches that the church should become involved in adjudicating a matter when someone refuses to deal with wrongdoing after private attempts at reconciliation do not succeed. However, the purpose remains reconciliation. A prime example lies in the situation in the church at Corinth. Paul rebuked the church for not disciplining a man who was having an immoral relationship.

Between First Corinthians and Second Corinthians, the Scripture shows how the church disciplined the person and put him out of the fellowship. The man repented and Paul instructed the church to receive him back into the church: "Sufficient to such a man is this punishment, which was inflicted of many. So that contrariwise you ought rather to forgive him, and comfort him, lest perhaps such a one should be swallowed up with overmuch sorrow. Wherefore I beseech you that you would confirm your love toward him. . . . Lest Satan should get an advantage of us: for we are not ignorant of his devices" (2 Corinthians 2:6–11).

Conflict is never fun. It hurts everyone involved and often inflicts collateral damage in the lives of others. Churches do not thrive when engaged in ongoing struggles. Families can disintegrate under the pressure of persistent conflict. Most of all, God's name is profaned when His children fight each other. For the sake of the church, our families, our own peace of mind, and the reputation of Christ, we have a responsibility to be peacemakers. As such, people will recognize us as God's children and glorify Him.

Chapter Nine

WHAT ABOUT THE GIANTS IN MY LIFE?

Handling Bullies

I have met my share of bullies through the years. You probably have too. They intimidate, threaten, shame, injure, and generally make life miserable—if you let them. Bullies come in all forms. When you were a child, you may have run into the kid who was bigger, older, stronger, and meaner—the one who pushed you around, stole your lunch money, and always wanted to fight. Or your bully could have been the girl who teased you, made jokes about you, and shamed you in front of others. The bully in your life may have been a teacher, parent, boss, or other adult whose words and actions hurt you deeply. I still remember an elementary school teacher who punished me by spanking me with a broom before putting me in the classroom trashcan and dumping trash on top of me while the class laughed. Just because someone has power does not mean it is right to use it abusively.

Adults also experience bullies, in the workplace, at home, around the neighborhood, and even in church. Victims of bullying often experience stress that affects many other areas of life. They become unmotivated at work, disconnect from church, and isolate themselves from the community. They appear sullen, angry, or discouraged. Adult casualties of bullying can suffer silently or strike out without warning and seemingly without reason.

Wounded people often wound others. They feel frustrated and helpless, so they sometimes launch their pain at others who are more vulnerable than themselves. Spouses, children, and even pets can become targets. Pressures build, stress mounts, and eventually the sufferers react—either toward others or against themselves. Betty was just such a person. She had been abused as a child. Her pain hid just beneath the surface of her emotions until they burst out in the form of violence against her children. They had become second-generation victims of the abusive bullying Betty had experienced. Her past did not excuse her actions, but the cycle of harm continued until Betty found help from an understanding pastor.

In milder situations, people may simply avoid the person causing them pain. Changes in schools, jobs, or churches provide temporary relief, but the sufferer usually discovers the new venue has its share of bullies too. If the situation is not resolved, or if it gets worse, the victim may seek a more extreme means of escape. Much too frequently we hear of another teenager who commits suicide or an adult who strikes out in violence.

The Bible recounts cases of bullies like Samson who intimidated and dominated his own parents, placing himself and his personal pleasure above them and the Lord (Judges 14:1–3). He attributed his great strength not to God, but to his hair, and in the end suffered painful humiliation before returning in repentance to the Lord.

Jezebel was perhaps the most infamous female bully of the Bible. Although the prophet Elijah had won a great victory over four hundred false prophets of a false god, he fled before the female fury of this wicked woman. Hiding in a mountain cave, he fell into depression and despondency, asking God to let him die (1 Kings 19–21).

Bullies Can Be Found Nearly Everywhere

At School

Children of all ages fall prey to bullies at school. Despite the best efforts of teachers and parents to eliminate the threat of intimidation, it still happens. On the school playground, one child may dominate the group because of physical size or willingness to injure others. Sometimes, the bully may be the child who is excluded from the group and fights back by hurting the weakest, most vulnerable classmate. In some worst-case scenarios, teachers may ignore or even encourage the kinds of competition that leads to bullying.

Upon reaching adolescence, the more mature bully does not grow out of harmful behavior but simply has more ways to push others around. The instrument of choice may be physical force or public shaming—either with unkind words or cyberbullying through social media. In extreme situations, actual weapons are brought to school, creating dangerous conditions that too often have resulted in injuries or even deaths. In some cases, the person wielding the knife or gun is someone who has been bullied and thinks the only way to respond is with more violence.

Parents should watch for signs of abuse related to their children or teens' school environment. They may frequently complain of illness or simply not want to go to school. Their grades suffer. Patterns of eating or sleeping may appear disrupted. They isolate themselves from peers or insulate themselves with the wrong crowd.

Some teens may start hanging around with groups, or even gangs, for self-protection and a sense of acceptance. Bobby found himself constantly bullied at his school. Older, stronger kids laughed at him, humiliated him in front of others, and finally started physically assaulting him on his way home from school. He found safety by joining a local gang. However, what small degree of security he gained was more than offset by the gang's demands that he join them in various criminal acts.

If children and teens know their parents are genuinely interested in their pain and have a sound relationship, they may share what is happening. However, mid-teens may believe that telling their parents about their problems is childish. They don't want to be known as "snitches" or unable to handle their own difficulties. Wanting to become more independent, teens often withdraw from the very family support that they need. All the while, the stress of daily pain continues unless the wise parent finds a way to break through the adolescent defense and connect with help and hope.

In the Family

Christian homes should be havens of security. Families ought to provide a safe environment of nurture. Children, teens, and adults look forward to coming home to people who accept and love them. Unfortunately, such is not always the case. Even Christian families can experience the pain of bullying. The perpetrators may not be genuinely saved, or they may be carnal in their spiritual nature; in any case, they inflict much stress and pain even on the best of families.

The father may abuse his wife and/or children either physically or verbally. Emotional attacks can produce just as much pain as physical injury. He may have learned such behavior growing up, or he might be acting out his own pain from a stressful situation at work. In either case, he has no excuse for wounding people who are in his care. Scripture warns about the evil man who "speaks froward things; who leaves the paths of uprightness to walk in the ways of darkness; who rejoices to do evil, and delights in the frowardness of the wicked, . . ." (Proverbs 2:12–14).

Sometimes, the wife may be the bully. Proverbs reminds us, "It is better to dwell in a corner of the housetop, than with a brawling woman in a wide house" (Proverbs 21:9). She may employ words instead of brute force, but is just as hurtful. She may lash out at her children with harsh words or physical force. There is something especially harmful when a mother's nature is to wound rather than heal. She may be expressing personal anger, frustration, or even self-loathing for some real or perceived issue of the past, yet the result is the same and remains without justification.

Siblings naturally experience a degree of rivalry as they grow up. However, a child or teen can become the bully of the family, dominating others by force of will or even physical abuse. Godly and wise parents should be sensitive to interactions between their children and teenagers. Observant adults can perceive emotional or relational changes that indicate a problem exists. Intervention involves protecting the vulnerable children from the bully and using biblical discipline to help the bully repent and change. Counseling may be necessary to help aggressive children or teens deal with their problems. Family love, prayer, and setting a good example can provide the foundation for forgiveness and healing.

In extreme cases, a spouse or child may need to find shelter outside the immediate family. The answer to an abusive spouse should not automatically default to divorce, but neither should the victim be forced to submit to further injury. Scriptural admonitions for a wife to submit herself to her husband (Ephesians 5:22) do not mean she is expected to subject herself or her children to physical abuse. A temporary relocation with family members or shelters can provide a safe environment while attempts are made to resolve the issues. If the mother is the abuser, the father may have to remove the children from her care while using legal and religious options, along with biblical counseling, to intervene with his wife.

Ultimately, the abuser may need to be confronted by civil authorities and/or the church to stop the bullying. Nearly all states have laws governing abuse—whether of a child, a spouse, or an elderly person in one's care. Not only do perpetrators face severe criminal penalties, people who know about such abuse are required by law to report the matter to appropriate authorities.

At Work

Laws governing the workplace usually give employees a stronger position when dealing with bullies on the job. Unfortunately, intimidation can be very subtle, but just as stressful. The source may be a coworker or someone holding the power over employment or promotions. A bullying coworker may be verbally abusive, throw work onto a colleague, or use innuendo and outright lies to undercut fellow workers. Supervisors generally want what's best for the business and the employee since they are under authority as well as in authority (Matthew 8:9). However, a bully with power in the workplace can rob workers of the joy of their jobs, add stress to their emotional load, and create an undercurrent of hostility.

At Church

The house of God should be a place of peace. We expect people identified with the Prince of Peace to get along with one another. In reality, conflict occurs in the church because people are people—some are not saved, others are carnal, but all wrestle with sin's legacy. Sadly, some churches suffer from an infestation of bullies. The perpetrator might be the pastor who thinks the church exists for his benefit.

More commonly, the church bully is a layperson who uses personal power to push other people around. Perhaps the aggressor has been a lifelong bully who simply applies in the church what works in other places. Matriarchs and patriarchs of significant families in the church wield control over others, including the pastor. Power can come through longevity in the church, financial influence, social status, or mere personal aggression. Most people who attend church go along to get along. Rather than engage in conflict, they simply let the bully have his or her way.

The New Testament Church was not ignorant of church bullies. John the Beloved Disciple wrote about Diotrephes who loved having preeminence in the church. He not only refused to receive John and other brothers but refused to allow the church to accept them. John recalled the "malicious words" Diotrephes used in an attempt to discredit the apostles. John declared that he would hold this man accountable for his actions (3 John 1:9–11). Similarly, the church must not let church bullies get away with their evil actions but should stand up to them and exercise discipline to bring them to repentance.

In the Community

Bullies can be found across your backyard fence, in civic organizations, and sitting on community boards. The bully may be the guy who berates the check-out clerk at the local store, the argumentative bore in the Parents-Teachers organization at your children's school, and the loud lady screaming at you because she didn't get her way in the community club.

Bullies Use a Variety of Weapons

Physical Threat

Children and teenagers tend to experience the intimidation of violence more often than adults. Usually the bully is larger physically, although some bullies are small, tough kids who threaten other children. Usually, adults are not present and the bully operates in the absence of the restraint of authority.

Words

The childhood rhyme is wrong: "Sticks and stones may break my bones, but words will never harm me." Words are harmful, often more so than physical violence. Broken bones can heal, but wounded spirits may be harder to mend. Children and teens can say cruel things to one another. As the child grows older, verbal cuts become sharper and the pain they inflict is more severe. Teenage girls especially tend to use damaging words to injure and control other girls.

Adult bullies also use sharpened tongues to injure others. The book of James warns about the harmful use of the tongue: "And the tongue is a fire, a world of iniquity: so is the tongue among our members, that it defiles the whole body, and sets on fire the course of nature; and it is set on fire of hell" (James 3:6).

Among the things God despises is the use of words to injure others. Listen to the words of the Wisdom Writer: "These six things does the LORD hate: yes, seven are an abomination to him: a proud look, a lying tongue, and hands that shed innocent blood, a heart that devises wicked imaginations, feet that are swift in running to mischief, a false witness that speaks lies, and he that sows discord among brothers" (Proverbs 6:16–19).

Shaming

Closely related to harmful words is the weapon of shame. A person who has done something wrong often feels shame and contrition. Shaming is something else entirely. Bullies who employ shame as a weapon do not rely on actual guilt but use matters over which the victim has little or no control. Using sarcasm, practical pranks, and public ridicule, the bully embarrasses the weaker person. The issue might be physical—making jokes about some aspect of the victim's appearance. It might be financial—degrading someone whose family does not have much money. The emotional attack can highlight a mistake that has been made, a lisp of the voice, or even the location of the victim's home (on the "other side of the tracks"). Proverbs describes ungodly people who dig up evil, sow strife, and separate friends. Such a person's lips are "as a burning fire" (Proverbs 16:27–28).

159

Cyberbullying

The advent of social media provides bullies with powerful weapons—wide accessibility and hidden anonymity. With a click of a computer key, someone can slay another's reputation, post embarrassing photos, or make false accusations that deeply wound the target. Scripture describes this kind of person: "He that hides hatred with lying lips and he that utters slander is a fool" (Proverbs 10:18).

Cindy was one example of the victims of cyberbullying. Other girls at her school put a series of humiliating posts about her on social media. With cruel lies and half-truths, they destroyed her reputation among her peers. Her friends became afraid to defend her or associate with her. She did not share her struggle with parents or teachers. She was isolated, afraid, hurt, and alone. This tragic result was not an isolated instance. Cyberbullying can deeply wound its victims.

Teenagers are not the only brunt of bullies who hide behind the Internet. One sad and dangerous reality in church life has been the use of the Internet by persons who launch attacks on their pastors. A number of pastors, particularly of larger churches, have been the objects of anonymous bloggers who can make accusations without offering substantiation. In many cases, the taint of wrongdoing adheres to the minister's reputation whether deserved or not.

Power of Position

Problems with abuse of positional power exist not only in the church or workplace but it can often be observed in the average social circle. Women especially find themselves vulnerable to the person who abuses their need for acceptance. Rather than find themselves the object of objectionable gossip, many women will yield to the social bully, providing the perpetrator with additional power. The author of Proverbs reminds us, "The words of a talebearer *are* as wounds, and they go down into the innermost parts of the belly" (Proverbs 18:8).

Men, on the other hand, tend to experience exploitation of authority in the workplace. Women, of course, also suffer job-related bullying, including sexual harassment. When an unscrupulous person gets into a place of power, the workplace becomes a tremendous source of stress.

Why Do People Put Up with Bullies?

Some victims are powerless. They may not be as strong physically or emotionally. Lacking the ability to fight back and unwilling or unable to flee, they endure the bully's attacks until they can find some way of escape.

Many sufferers put up with the problem for other reasons. People of all ages want to be accepted. Victims may endure the constant pain imposed by the bully in order to be accepted, sometimes by the injurious person or by a group that person controls.

Similarly, wives who feel they need the financial or emotional support of an abusive husband may defend and excuse his actions. A few may even overlook husbands' abuse of their children because they feel they have no alternative. Husbands who have abusive spouses can experience similar situations, but for different reasons. Many sufferers don't believe in divorce, so they stoically endure and silently suffer.

Don't Let Bullies Own You or Your Future

You can run, but you cannot hide. Bullies are everywhere. Rather than letting them crush your contentment, learn to respond effectively and biblically.

Resist

Most bullies are cowards at heart. They push people around because no one stands up to them. Often, when confronted, they back down and, sometimes, leave their targets alone. You might ask, "What about turning the other cheek and going the other mile?" Jesus' admonition in Matthew 5:38 warns against seeking revenge: "an eye for an eye, a tooth for a tooth." Resisting is not revenge. Godly resistance is a demonstration of godly love. Love does not allow a bully to continue hurting people. In truth, bullies are hurting themselves. True love stops them.

Tommy had been pushed around physically and verbally for several years. His primary antagonist, John, looked for any opportunity to attack him. John usually used situations in which Tommy could not fight back.

Finally, Tommy stood up to John in front of several peers. Confronted publically, John backed down and stopped bullying Tommy. I do not advocate violence, but unless bullies are resisted in a proper way, they generally continue their aggression.

Rebuke

Scripture consistently urges us to rebuke people who are doing wrong. "If a brother trespass against you, rebuke him; and if he repent, forgive him" (Luke 17:3). Often, we focus on the forgiveness aspect of our duty to others and overlook the responsibility we have to rebuke offenders.

At the same time, understand that foolish people often respond to godly rebuke in unkind ways. Brutish people hate reproof (Proverbs 12:1). The bully may initially respond with vengeful words or actions (Proverbs 9:7–8).

Still, true love casts out fear (1 John 4:18), so you should not be afraid to confront someone who has injured you or others through bullying. You will probably have to take the initiative in correcting the offender since bullies seldom feel remorseful for their offenses. Be humble but firm when dealing with someone who has hurt you (Galatians 6:1).

Pray and Do Good

Jesus urged His followers to pray for their enemies, even those who "despitefully use you and persecute you" (Matthew 5:44). Prayer is a demonstration of godly love. Proof of loving prayer is demonstrated by doing good to people who hurt us. Again, praying for someone and doing good to an enemy does not mean you are approving his or her actions. Instead, you are seeking God's best by desiring that person see Christ in you and, hopefully, bringing the individual to the Lord Who can change lives for the better.

Protect

Godly people have a duty to protect the weaker brother and sister (or son and daughter) from anyone who would do injury to them. We are called on to defend people who are powerless to help themselves. Psalm 82:3 instructs us to "defend the poor and fatherless: do justice to the afflicted and needy." Sometimes that means to intervene physically to prevent harm coming to someone. It could require verbal intercession. Involvement of legal authorities may be necessary.

In the church, for the good of the Body of Christ and its testimony to the lost, bullies cannot be tolerated. Church discipline is one way to deal with the church bully. Remember, the goal is to restore the wrongdoer, so the initial approach should always be personal and humble, with the hope that the person will repent and behave differently. However, if unrepentant and repetitive in their aggression, bullies should be treated like nonbelievers and be removed from the church's fellowship (Matthew 18:15–17).

Gossips are verbal bullies. Strife always follows in the wake of a talebearer's tongue. "The words of a talebearer are as wounds, and they go down into the innermost parts of the belly" (Proverbs 26:22). Sometimes the only way to bring harmony and unity to any group, including the church, is to remove the source of the conflict. Proverbs offers sound wisdom at this point: "Where no wood is, there the fire goes out: so where there is no talebearer, the strife ceases. As coals are to burning coals, and wood to fire; so is a contentious man to kindle strife" (Proverbs 26:20–21).

Maintain Faith and Hope

Even in tribulation, we have access by faith into God's grace and can stand steadfastly in the hope of God. Remember that "tribulation works patience; and patience, experience; and experience, hope: and hope makes (us) not ashamed; because the love of God is shed abroad in our hearts by the Holy Ghost which is given unto us" (Romans 5:3–5).

Through it All, Don't Get Bitter

Trust the Lord to give you the strength and wisdom to respond correctly to bullies. Remember, the bully cannot define who you are. Your identity, worth, and purpose are found in Christ. His Spirit living in you can give you the victory even under persecution. Paul taught his son in the gospel, Timothy, that all who live godly lives will suffer persecution

(2 Timothy 3:12). We should not find it strange that wicked people will attack us. At the same time, we need to be sure we are not being targeted because we have done something wrong (1 Peter 4:12–17).

As someone has said, instead of getting bitter, get better. Heed Peter's encouragement: "And beside this, giving all diligence, add to your faith virtue; and to virtue knowledge; and to knowledge temperance; and to temperance patience; and to patience godliness; and to godliness brotherly kindness; and to brotherly kindness charity. For if these things be in you, and abound, they make you that ye shall neither be barren nor unfruitful in the knowledge of our Lord Jesus Christ" (2 Peter 1:5–8).

Chapter Ten
WHAT ABOUT SPECIAL CASES?

Extreme Stress: Burnout and PTSD

S uper stress. Burnout and PTSD are stress on steroids. Burnout is not as common as one might think, but when someone reaches this degree of unmanaged stress, strong measures should be taken to survive. Post-Traumatic Stress Disorder (PTSD) is also more discussed than experienced. Many people go through traumatic experiences, whether in war or violent crime, without falling prey to PTSD's insidious effects. Still, both conditions are very real and can be very dangerous.

Christian families are not immune to either condition. The good news for them and others is both problems can be overcome. Just as severe medical problems can be conquered with the correct treatment, even so believers can find healing from burnout and PTSD.

What follows is not medical or psychological advice but observations and spiritual principles that offer hope to sufferers of each problem. Persons who believe they are experiencing either of these conditions should also seek competent help from appropriate Christian counselors or physicians. These few pages cannot offer comprehensive analysis of either issue. They are intended to provide spiritual insights and, most of all, hope.

Surviving Burnout

When stress continues unabated and unmanaged, burnout inevitably follows. This tertiary level of stress has been termed *exhaustion*.

Most believers who reach this stage have strong enough spiritual commitment to avoid destructive responses. Still, many sufferers merely trudge through each day, feeling hopeless. Without help and spiritual renewal, many Christians who remain at the burnout stage long enough will resort to poor choices that hurt themselves and others.

Evidence of Burnout

Burnout may manifest itself in depression, inability to engage in normal activities and responsibilities, lack of care for oneself and others, and a desire to escape. Some sufferers spend inordinate time in bed, trying to escape into sleep with the aid of whatever sedatives are available. Others may simply walk away, either from their jobs, their families, or both. A few escape life itself through suicide.

Glen Martin, in his book *Beyond the Rat Race*, describes several warning signs of stress overload: emotional and mental fatigue evidenced in constant feelings of discouragement, inability to enjoy life, impatience, perfectionism, spiritual disinterest, problems with relationships, and inappropriate priorities.[1]

Causes of Burnout

One of the most common causes of burnout involves focusing on the task to the exclusion of spiritual development. Without spiritual renewal and adopting proper priorities, Christians can keep giving without taking in until they have nothing left for themselves or others. One study observed that burnout among workaholics is inevitable, especially if people base their self-esteem on productivity.[2]

An obvious contributor to burnout is sin. When we are out of God's will, we open ourselves up to spiritual attack from without and within. Satan's minions accuse us and we wallow in guilt. More importantly, God's Spirit brings conviction into the hearts of His children to draw them to repentance. Although he was the king of Israel and a man after God's heart, David reached that point. His story in Psalm 32 described how he arrived at the point where his bones seemed so brittle as to break and his strength was dried up within him. He spent all day groaning in misery (Psalm 32:3–4).

Ultimately, we could revisit all the various causes of stress because burnout can trace its roots to each of them. Whenever we experience sufficiently high levels of unmanaged stress over long periods of time, we are susceptible to burnout.

Effects on the Family

When parents suffer burnout, the entire family experiences the effects. Children see Mom or Dad going through this unusual change and feel threatened. The father may normally play or otherwise interact with his kids, but now he comes home and avoids them. He may have been fun; now he mopes around the house often showing little or no emotion. As children watch their mom expend extra time and energy to help fill the gap, they may become angry at their parents.

Family Burnout

Family members are also susceptible to burnout. Burnout can strike anyone. Wives have their own challenges from persistent, pervasive stress. One study of over three hundred women revealed a strong correlation between burnout and incessantly trying to live up to everyone's expectations. From their study, Sue Eenigenburg and Robynn Bliss observed that not only does the woman have expectations of herself that may be unrealistic, but she also perceives strong expectations from her spouse and family, coworkers, and neighbors.[3] Trying to live up to unrealistic expectations can produce unhealthy attempts at perfectionism, which is unattainable in this life. Strong inner forces can drive sufferers beyond the brink of burnout.

In addition, women experience pain as they watch their husbands undergo distress. In some cases, spouses can become codependent along with their husbands. They enjoy being needed, while at the same time they are stressed by the caring process.

Children undergo their own sources of stress overload. Sometimes the parents are too caught up in their responsibilities, and perhaps their own levels of burnout, and they don't notice the pain their kids are experiencing. Keeping vigil over children is the responsibility of the entire family. Watch for signs of unusual lethargy, the lack of normal emotions, not wanting to engage in play with friends, and growing ambivalence toward activities that formerly generated excitement. Major changes of habits regarding eating and sleeping may also be evidence of abnormal stress. Parents would be wise to consult physicians, since the child may need medical care, as each problem could be a symptom of physical ailments.

Recovery from Burnout

The term *burnout* seems to leave little hope. The word bears the image of someone so totally empty as to be irretrievably lost. Don't believe it! God does not leave his pilgrims in the "slough of despond," as John Bunyan described what we might call spiritual depression. Our heavenly Father is able to heal, renew, and revitalize His children. God can heal in an instant, or He may choose to initiate recovery involving a number of steps:

Recognition. One of the first steps to overcoming burnout is to acknowledge you are experiencing it. Ministers may sense shame for not living up to what may be unrealistic expectations. Realize that godly people have gone through similar feelings. Moses came to the point of frustration and fatigue that he asked God to let him die (Numbers 11:14–15). After a miraculous victory over the prophets of Baal, Elijah was persecuted by Jezebel. In his flight, he prayed that God would take his life (1 Kings 19:1–18). In both cases, God intervened and restored both to effective ministry. Christians should not be embarrassed or feel any sense of failure if they reach this level of stress. Greater men and women than they have suffered similarly. Their stories should encourage us to appraise our situation honestly and humbly seek help from the Great Physician.

Reconnecting. Brooks Faulkner recommends a comprehensive program of defeating burnout, including attacking the problem on personal, professional, physical, and other levels. Coping strategies include reestablishing proper priorities, allowing intervention from peers and professionals, and seeking divine help from the Lord.[4] Maintaining freedom from burnout can be more successful with a network of support, including family, friends, and professional counselors.

Sufferers should not shy away from seeking legitimate medical help. This recommendation does not suggest finding some pill to alleviate the symptoms alone. Rather, recognize that the exhaustion level of stress affects the body. A thorough physical can reveal if underlying medical problems, illnesses, or even cancer may be at the root of the various symptoms.

Renewal. Recognizing the brokenness in one's life, the next step to restoration is personal spiritual renewal. As with other problems, people experiencing burnout need healing that only God can supply. Part of their problem includes their inability or unwillingness to appropriate the power of the Lord. They may harbor sin that they are unwilling to resolve through repentance and forgiveness. They likely have ceased regular communion with Christ in prayer and scriptural meditation. Donald Demaray observes, "Healing can only take place when imbedded sin comes to the surface to be cleansed away. . . . The penitent sinner finds immense release."[5]

Reach out to God. Sometimes, burnout victims may be under such extreme exhaustion they are unable to do anything more than call out to God for help. He loves us and understands exactly where we are. He hears our cries and responds. The children of Israel cried to God in their distress and He responded with a deliverer—Moses (Exodus 2:23). When Israel came under persecution during the days of judges, the people cried out to God Who sent a rescuer (Judges 3:9).

Do you feel weak and helpless? God spoke of such people in terms of widows and orphans when He promised: "If thou afflict them in any wise, and they cry at all unto me, I will surely hear their cry" (Exodus 22:23). A Canaanite woman cried out to Jesus on behalf of her demonized daughter, and the ultimate Deliverer responded (Matthew 15:22ff). Even so, cry out to the Lord. He hears and responds with deliverance and healing.

Coping with Post-Traumatic Stress

In a fallen world, people face dangers on a regular basis. Terrorism, violent crime, home invasions, carjacking, kidnapping, and other traumatic experiences befall average people who are simply trying to live quiet lives. One of the consequences can be post-traumatic stress. Christians are not exempt from this form of extreme strain. We need to recognize its symptoms and take steps to deal with it.

PTSD Reactions

People who suffer severe trauma experience immediate stress reactions, and they often have flashbacks, fear, anxiety, or other symptoms long after the crisis has passed. The Mayo Clinic identifies PTSD symptoms. Some victims experience flashbacks or nightmares in which the trauma is relived. Others may express unwillingness to talk about the trauma even to the point of avoiding friends who want to help. They may be easily startled or seem jumpy. They may present a sense of helplessness and hopelessness. They may have trouble sleeping, feel restless, and express unexpected bursts of anger. Normal emotions may seem blunted as the sufferer falls into a depressive lethargy. They may begin using various medications.[6]

Children and PTSD

Children often take more time to work through trauma than do adults. Charlesworth and Nathan observe: "They will withdraw, or, conversely, chatter about everything except the event until they feel safe enough to talk about the trauma. They may take even longer if there is no one whom they trust to reach out to them with sensitivity and patience to get them to talk about the event or act it out in play or artwork."[7] The National Institute for Mental Health warns that children who may suffer from PTSD might relapse into bed-wetting. They may constantly cling physically and emotionally to one or both parents and feel panic when separated.[8]

Responding to PTSD

Secular organizations, such as the National Institute for Mental Health and the Veterans Administration, focus on various methods of counseling, medications, and other treatments for PTSD sufferers. Certainly, victims should seek competent counsel, but believers will want to consult qualified Christian counselors who employ methods based on biblical principles. Whether certain medications are needed should be determined by physicians who take time to understand the spiritual, mental, and emotional aspects of the problem. Use of tranquilizers or antidepressants has come under increased scrutiny by such agencies as the NIMH. This writing is not intended to discourage proper medication but rather encourages believers to seek counselors and doctors who share common values.

Family and friends can also help PTSD victims, often simply by being available. Don't demand that the persons talk, but be present if they want to discuss their feelings. Someone who has gone through some type of traumatic experience and recovered often provides a familiar, safe relationship in which victims can open up. The more the sufferers can verbalize their fears and talk about their experience, the sooner they can overcome its effects.

Families affected by crisis or trauma find mutual support in one another through prayer and practical means. The ministry of presence, just being there for one another, provides vital encouragement. Affected families often need help with basic needs, including food preparation, help with the children, and assistance with ministry responsibilities.

Parents naturally give prime attention to supporting their children during crises. At the same time, they have to manage their own emotions. While adults try to remain strong for their children's sake, they need the freedom to express their feelings to one another. Delaying venting of emotions can set them up for post-traumatic stress disorder later. Competent counselors and compassionate friends offer safe harbors where fears, hurts, and other reactions can be shared.

Through every trial, believers' best comfort is the triune God Whom they serve. We have a heavenly Father Who cares about each pain and hears every prayer. Our Savior, Jesus, intercedes for us at the right hand of the Father with the understanding of One Who suffered for us. The blessed Holy Spirit is a Divine Comforter Who comes alongside to strengthen and console us. With God's help, Christian families can endure and experience healing.

CONCLUSION: HOPE!

S tress is part of life. Believers cannot opt out of stress, but we can equip ourselves to cope and overcome. God gives His children wonderful spiritual resources to help handle whatever comes our way, including stressful situations.

Christ's Body, the Church, provides a welcoming fellowship of brothers and sisters with diverse backgrounds, experiences, and abilities. Within the church we support each other, pray for one another, and contribute to each other's well-being.

God's Word includes amazing principles for life. Following God's precepts results in harmony and direction with God's purpose for our lives. Scripture guides our marriages and families, enhances our relationships with people, and helps us know Him.

The Holy Spirit actually lives inside the believer's spirit, bearing witness that we are God's children. He glorifies Jesus, convicts us of sin, intercedes with us in prayer, empowers us with His spiritual gifts, and produces His fruit in our lives.

Jesus, God the Son, loved us and laid down His life for us. He conquered death that we might have eternal and abundant life. He stands today ever living to make intercession for us. He is coming again to receive us to Himself so that where He is we can also be.

God, the heavenly Father, before He ever created us or a world to live in, saw our need for a Savior and fashioned an eternal plan none of us could imagine. "For God so loved the world that He gave His only begotten Son, that whosoever believes in Him should not perish but have everlasting life" (John 3:16). He is holy, majestic, all powerful, all knowing, always present, and He wants us to have a personal relationship with Him through faith in His Son. Amazing!

With a God like that, we can face life with confidence and hope. We can experience lives of joy and abundance. We can overcome stress and anything else life throws at us, "For I am persuaded, that neither death, nor life, nor angels, nor principalities, nor powers, nor things present, nor things to come, nor height, nor depth, nor any other creature, shall be able to separate us from the love of God, which is in Christ Jesus our Lord" (Romans 8:38–39).

ENDNOTES

Chapter One

1. None of the names used in this work reflect actual identities of individuals.

Chapter Two

1. Hans Selye, *Stress Without Distress* (New York: Signet, 1975
2. cf. National Institute of Health, http://www.ncbi.nlm.nih.gov/pmc/articles/PMC2153803/
3. Charles Solomon, *Handbook to Happiness* (Wheaton: Tyndale House, 1986), 38.
4. American Medical Association, Charles Clayman, M.D., ed. *Family Medical Guide* (New York: Random House, 1994), 38.
5. Scott Litin, M.D., *The Mayo Clinic Family Health Book*, 4th ed. (Rochester, Minn: Mayo Clinic, 2009), 291–292.
6. Donald Demaray, *Watch Out for Burnout* (Grand Rapids: Baker, 1983), 14.
7. Litin, 293.
8. Referenced in Kevin Leman, *The 6 Stress Points in a Woman's Life* (Grand Rapids: Fleming Revell, 1999), 34.
9. Taylor-Johnson Temperament Analysis (Thousand Oaks, California: Psychological Publications, Inc.).
10. Tim LaHaye, *Spirit-Controlled Temperament* (New York: Tyndale House, 1966).

Chapter Three

1. William Shakespeare, "Julius Caesar," Act 2, Scene 2.

Chapter Four

1. Martin Lloyd-Jones, *Spiritual Depression*. Grand Rapids: Eerdmans, 1965.
2. William Shakespeare, "Measure for Measure," Act 1, Scene 4.

Chapter Five

1. Solomon, 50ff.
2. Bill Bright, "Have you made the wonderful discovery of the Spirit-filled life?" Campus Crusade for Christ.
3. Hannah Whitehall Smith, *The Christian's Secret of a Happy Life* (New York: Fleming Revell, 1952), 46–47.
4. Ibid., 37.
5. Andrew Murray, *A Life of Obedience* (Minneapolis: Bethany House, 2004), 71.
6. Johnson Oatman, Jr., "Count Your Many Blessings," 1897, public domain.
7. Solomon, 44–45. (For a good study of this subject, see Charles Solomon, *The Rejection Syndrome.* Wheaton: Tyndale House, 1988.)
8. Jay Adams, *Competent to Counsel* (Grand Rapids: Zondervan, 1970), 143.
9. Ibid., 93.
10. Richard Swenson, *Margin: Restoring Emotional, Physical, Financial, and Time Reserves to Overloaded Lives* (Colorado Springs: NavPress, 2004).
11. Martha Davis, Elizabeth Eshelman, and Matthew McKay, *The Relaxation and Stress Reduction Workbook* (New York: MUF Books, 1995), 35.

Chapter Six

1. John White, Parents in Pain: Overcoming the Hurt and Frustration of Problem Children (Downer's Grove: InterVarsity Press, 1979), 104.
2. Ruth Bell Graham, Prodigals and Those Who Love Them (Grand Rapids: Baker, 1999), 11.
3. Richard Burr, Praying Your Prodigal Home (Camp Hill, Penn.: Wing Spread Publishers, 2003), 80ff.
4. Ibid.
5. Quin Sherrer and Ruthanne Garlock, Praying Prodigals Home (Ventra, California: Regal, 2000).

Chapter Ten

1. Glen Martin, *Beyond the Rat Race* (Nashville: B&H, 1995), 13–21.
2. Echerd, 172.
3. Sue Eenigenburg and Robynn Bliss, *Expectations and Burnout: Women Surviving the Great Commission* (Pasadena, William Carey Library, 2010).
4. Brooks Faukner, *Burnout in Ministry* (Nashville: Broadman Press, 1981), 118 ff.
5. Donald Demaray, *Watch Out for Burnout* (Grand Rapids: Baker, 1983), 26.
6. Mayo Clinic, "Post-traumatic Stress Disorder," http://www.mayoclinic.com/health/post-traumatic-stress-disorder/DS00246/DSECTION=symptoms
7. Edward Charlesworth, Ph.D. and Ronald Nathan, Ph.D. *Stress Management: A Comprehensive Guide to Wellness* (New York: Ballantine Books, 2004), 15.
8. National Institute of Mental Health, "Post-traumatic Stress Disorder," http://www.nimh.nih.gov/health/topics/post-traumatic-stress-disorder-ptsd/index.shtml

BIBLIOGRAPHY

Abramowitz, Jonathan. *The Stressless Workbook*. New York: Guilford Press, 2012.

Adams, Jay. *Competent to Counsel*. Philipsburg, N.J.: Presbyterian and Reformed Publishing Co, 1970.

American Medical Association, Charles Clayman, M.D., ed. *Family Medical Guide*. New York: Random House, 1994.

Brandt, Henry and Kerry Skinner. *The Word for the Wise*. Nashville: B & H Publishers, 1995.

Brent, Caroline. *The Caregiver's Companion*. Harlequin: 2015.

Bright, Bill. "Have you made the wonderful discovery of the Spirit-filled life?" booklet, Campus Crusade for Christ.

Brown, Joe. *Battle Fatigue*. Nashville: B&H Publishers, 1995.

Burr, Richard. *Praying Your Prodigal Home*. Camp Hill, Penn: Wing Spread Publishers, 2003,

Charlesworth, Edward, Ph.D. and Ronald Nathan, Ph.D. *Stress Management: A Comprehensive Guide to Wellness*. New York: Ballentine Books, 2004.

Cohen-Sandler, Roni. *Stressed Out Girls: Helping Them Thrive in the Age of Pressure*. New York: Penguin, 2005.

Crabb, Larry. *Effective Biblical Counseling*. Grand Rapids: Zondervan, 1977.

David, Martha, Elizabeth Eshelman, and Matthew McKay. *The Relaxation and Stress Reduction Workbook*. New York: MUF Books, 1995.

Demaray, Donald. *Watch Out for Burnout*. Grand Rapids: Baker, 1983.

Echerd, Pam and Alice Arathoon, ed. *Understanding and Nurturing the Missionary Family*. Pasadena, Cal.: William Carey Library, 1989.

Eenigenburg Sue and Robynn Bliss, *Expectations and Burnout: Women Surviving the Great Commission*. Pasadena, William Carey Library, 2010.

Eliot, Robert S., M.D. *From Stress to Strength*. New York: Bantam Books, 1994.

England, Diane. *The Post-Traumatic Stress Disorder Relationship*. Avon, Mass.: Adams, 2009.

Ferrara, Miranda, ed. *Human Diseases and Conditions*, vol. 4. New York: Charles Scribers Sons, 2010.

Graham, Ruth Bell. *Prodigals and Those Who Love Them*. Grand Rapids: Baker, 1999.

Harris, Roy. *Caring for the Caregiver*. Tate Publishing, 2009.

Haugk, Kenneth C. *Christian Caregiving*. Minneapolis: Augsburg, 1984.

Huggins, Kevin. *Parenting Adolescents*. Colorado Springs: NavPress, 1989.

Lawson, Steven. *Faith Under Fire*. Wheaton: Crossway, 1995.

Lloyd-Jones, Martin. *Spiritual Depression*. Grand Rapids: Eerdmans, 1965.

LaHaye, Tim. *Spirit-Controlled Temperament*. New York: Tyndale House, 1966.

Lawson, Steven. *Faith Under Fire*. Wheaton: Crossway, 1995.

Litin, Scott, M.D. *The Mayo Clinic Family Health Book*, 4th ed. Rochester, Minn: Mayo Clinic, 2009.

Leman, Kevin. *The 6 Stress Points in a Woman's Life*. Grand Rapids: Fleming Revell, 1999.

Margolia, Simeon, M. D. *The John Hopkins Medical Guide to Health After 50*. New York: Rebus, 2002.

Martin, Glen *Beyond the Rat Race*. Nashville: B&H, 1995.

Murray, Andrew. *A Life of Obedience*. Minneapolis: Bethany House, 2004.

Oliver, Suzannah. *Stress Protection Plan*. London: Collins and Brown, 2000.

Rankin, Jerry. *Spiritual Warfare*. Nashville, B&H, 2009.

Richard, Ramesh. *Mending Your Soul*. Nashville: B&H, 1999.

Rush, Myron, *Management: A Biblical Approach*. Victor Books: 1983.

Scott, Buddy. *Relief for Hurting Parents*. Nashville: Oliver-Nelson Books, 1989.

Selye, Hans. *Stress Without Distress*. New York: Lippincott Williams & Wilkins, 1974.

Sherrer, Quin and Ruthanne Garlock, *Praying Prodigals Home*. Ventra, California: Regal, 2000.

Smalley, Gary. *The Key to Your Child's Heart*. Waco: Word, 1984.

Smith, Hannah Whitehall. *The Christian's Secret of a Happy Life*. New York: Fleming Revell, 1952.

Solomon, Charles. *Handbook to Happiness*. Wheaton: Tyndale House, 1999.

Swenson, Richard. *Margin: Restoring Emotional, Physical, Financial, and Time Reserves to Overloaded Lives.* Colorado Springs: NavPress, 2004.

White, John. *Parents in Pain: Overcoming the Hurt and Frustration of Problem Children.* Downer's Grove: InterVarsity Press, 1979.

Made in the USA
Coppell, TX
21 May 2020

26119702R00105